Fit to be Well

ESSENTIAL CONCEPTS

Fit to be Well

ESSENTIAL CONCEPTS

Alton L. Thygerson
Brigham Young University

JONES AND BARTLETT PUBLISHERS

Sudbury, Massachusetts

BOSTON   TORONTO   LONDON   SINGAPORE

World Headquarters

Jones and Bartlett Publishers
40 Tall Pine Drive
Sudbury, MA 01776
978-443-5000
info@jbpub.com
www.jbpub.com

Jones and Bartlett Publishers
Canada
2406 Nikanna Road
Mississauga, ON L5C 2W6
CANADA

Jones and Bartlett Publishers
International
Barb House, Barb Mews
London W6 7PA
UK

Production Credits

Chief Executive Officer: Clayton Jones
Chief Operating Officer: Don W. Jones, Jr.
President of Higher Education and
 Professional Publishing: Robert W. Holland, Jr.
V.P., Design and Production: Anne Spencer
V.P., Manufacturing and Inventory Control: Therese Bräuer
V.P., Sales and Marketing: William J. Kane
Acquisitions Editor: Jacqueline Ann Mark
Senior Production Editor: Julie Champagne Bolduc
Assistant Editor: Nicole Quinn
Editorial Assistant: Erin Murphy
Senior Marketing Manager: Ed McKenna
Director of Interactive Technology: Adam Alboyadjian
Interactive Technology Manager: Dawn Mahon Priest
Composition: Graphic World
Cover and Interior Design: Anne Spencer
Cover Image: © image100/Alamy Images
Printing and Binding: Courier Kendallville
Cover Printing: Courier Kendallville

Library of Congress Cataloging-in-Publication Data
Thygerson, Alton L.
 Fit to be well : essential concepts / Alton L. Thygerson.
 p. cm.
Includes bibliographical references and index.
ISBN 0-7637-2450-5
1. Health. 2. Physical fitness. I. Title.
RA776.T539 2005
613—dc22
        2004022990

Printed in the United States of America
09 08 07 06 05 10 9 8 7 6 5 4 3 2 1

Contents

CHAPTER ⑤ **Increasing Muscular Strength and
Endurance 64**

CHAPTER (6) **Choosing a Nutritious Diet 84**

CHAPTER **Assessing Body Composition 118**

CHAPTER 8 **Maintaining a Healthy Body Composition and Body Weight** 130

CHAPTER ⑨ **Managing Stress 150**

CHAPTER 10 Responsible Decision Making 168

The purposes of this book are, first, to introduce you to the extraordinary world of physical fitness, and second, to change your life.

In a time of high-tech advances, we have lost sight of the fact that the greatest high-tech invention of all time is the human body. What happens to our packaging—our bodies—as we move through life is the result of our lifestyle.

As priceless as good health is, it is paradoxically freely available to us, if we live the right way. The child does not have to be taught to play, but the adult must learn how to exercise. Adults lose that childhood instinct to run and jump, to skip, and to walk briskly. But it is movement, in assorted styles and speeds, on a regular basis, that is critical in maintaining our high-tech machinery.

The best news is that it is never too late to start exercising, eating properly, and managing stress, regardless of your age or physical condition. This book can help you to make those changes that will sustain your health, and therefore, make your life a better one.

Attempting to reach the goal of good health and wellness through physical fitness can be compared with preparing to take a journey. If you were driving from Los Angeles to New York City, you would first obtain a road map in order to determine the best route to follow. The journey to good health and wellness is very similar, but most people are not familiar with, or do not know where to obtain, a road map leading to good health and wellness.

This book represents such a road map. It takes you from your current level of fitness toward increased cardiorespiratory endurance, strength, and flexibility, as well as helping you to maintain a healthy weight and learn to relax.

Fit to be Well offers a simple, workable approach to a healthy lifestyle.

Note to Students and Instructors

No other fitness book is like this one, despite sharing similar content.
The content of this book is organized in a succinct, easy-to-navigate manner, with emphasis placed on important concepts and applications. The advantages of this approach include:

- Decreased reading time
- Quicker access to information
- Improved learning
- Less expensive
- High reader satisfaction
- Creative uses of information (e.g., uses "chunking" to put content into manageable units for better learning)
- No long-winded passages—the content is concise, straightforward information that a person "needs" to know rather than being "nice" to know.
- Evidence-based medical sources provide the content and latest recommendations.

Special Features

Special features to improve learning include:

What's the word...
Boxes throughout the text containing target terms offer simple, clear definitions to words of interest.

The Inside Track

Here you will find quick and easy guides to important information.

Tipping Point

These are helpful hints and tips on how to manage your fitness and healthy lifestyle program.

Knowledge Check

Multiple-choice questions appear at the end of each chapter to test your knowledge of the information covered in the text.

Modern Modifications

In each chapter there is a section that provides a list of simple suggestions related to that chapter's topic. Each of these suggestions are specifically intended to be easily absorbed into your daily routine. They are realistic and take into consideration "real life" obstacles.

Critical Thinking

These sections give you a chance to test what you learned in each chapter. Questions and scenarios about the work that you will do and the goals to achieve will bring about some critical thoughts. This will help you assimilate what you learn and apply it to your daily life.

Going Above and Beyond

At the end of each chapter, this book provides a perfect opportunity for those with a desire to take their research one step further. Complete bibliographies and websites are included so that you can take any of the information you find interesting and learn more.

Acknowledgments

Any book requires a great deal of effort, and not just on the part of the author. This book is no exception to that rule.

I am fortunate to have a publisher, Clayton Jones, who believes in this unique project, and who encouraged me to write this textbook. I am very grateful to Jacqueline Mark, acquisitions editor, for pushing the project along the way, and Erin Murphy for helping to make it a better book. A strong appreciation goes to the Jones and Bartlett Publishers production staff, including Anne Spencer and Julie Bolduc, for publishing a book of high quality, and to Graphic World for putting it all together.

To all of the reviewers, I express my thanks for their help and many worthwhile suggestions. Finally, I thank my wife for her encouragement and support.

Although there are no sure-fire recipes for good health, the mixture of regular exercise and healthy eating comes awfully close. According to the *New England Journal of Medicine* (Myers et al. 2002), poor physical fitness is a better predictor of death than smoking, hypertension, and heart disease. Although tobacco is still the top cause of avoidable deaths, the widespread pattern of physical inactivity combined with unhealthful diets is poised to top the list because of the resulting epidemic of obesity **Figure 1** (Mokdad et al. 2004). Americans are sitting around and eating themselves to death, with obesity closing in on tobacco as the nation's leading underlying preventable killer. The alarming part is that behavior is going in the wrong direction.

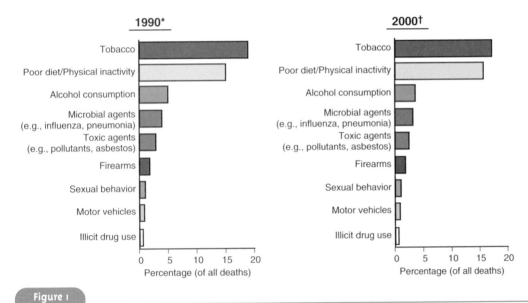

Figure 1

Comparing actual causes of death in the United States from 1990 to 2000. (Sources: * McGinnis, J.M. and Foege, W.H. *Journal of the American Medical Association.* 1993; 270(18):2207-2212; † Mokdad, A., Marks, J., Stroup D., and Gerberding, J. Actual causes of death in the United States, 2000. *Journal of the American Medical Association.* March 10, 2004;291:1238-1245.

Regular exercise, or physical activity, can do everyone a world of good. It helps prevent heart disease, diabetes, osteoporosis, and a host of other diseases, and is a key ingredient for losing weight or maintaining a healthy weight.

With all these advantages, it is mind boggling that only a minority of Americans get enough exercise or leisure-time physical activity to benefit them. Studies that have followed the health of large groups of people for many years, as well as short-term studies of the physiologic effects of exercise, all point in the same direction: *A sedentary (inactive) lifestyle increases the chances of becoming overweight and developing a number of chronic diseases.*

Exercise or regular physical activity helps many of the body's systems function better and keeps a host of diseases at bay.

According to the U.S. Surgeon General's report, *Physical Activity and Health* (U.S. Department of Health and Human Services 1996) regular physical activity:

- Improves your chances of living longer and living healthier
- Helps protect you from developing heart disease and its precursors, high blood pressure and high cholesterol

- Helps protect you from developing certain cancers, including colon and breast cancer
- Helps prevent or control type 2 diabetes (previously called adult-onset diabetes)
- Helps prevent arthritis and may relieve pain and stiffness in people with this condition
- Helps prevent the insidious loss of bone known as osteoporosis
- Reduces the risk of falling among older adults
- Controls weight

If you do not currently exercise and are not very active during the day, any increase in exercise or physical activity is good for you. Some studies show that walking briskly for even one to two hours a week (15 to 20 minutes a day) starts to decrease the chances of having a heart attack or stroke, developing diabetes, or dying prematurely.

Definitions

The following terms will help to get you started toward a vocabulary of good health.

Health The 1946 World Health Organization's definition of health has been used as a foundation for the contemporary term of wellness (WHO 1946). "Health is a state of complete physical, mental, and social well-being and not merely the absence of disease or infirmity."

Wellness There are many definitions of wellness. All definitions focus on the nature of personal responsibility as being a key to wellness. The National Wellness Institute offers that wellness is an active process of becoming aware of and making choices toward a more successful existence. Wellness is multidimensional consisting of six dimensions: (1) social, (2) occupational, (3) spiritual, (4) physical, (5) intellectual, and (6) emotional.

Physical activity Bodily movement produced by skeletal muscles that increases energy expenditure.

Exercise Planned, structured, and repetitive physical activity done to improve or maintain one or more components of physical fitness.

Physical fitness Set of attributes that people have or achieve that relates to the ability to perform physical activity. Health-related components of physical fitness include:

- Cardiorespiratory endurance
- Muscular strength
- Muscular endurance
- Flexibility
- Body composition

National Wellness Goals

The U.S. DHHS launched *Healthy People 2010* (2000), a comprehensive, nationwide health promotion and disease prevention agenda. *Healthy People 2010* serves as a road map for improving the health of all people in the United States during the first decade of the 21st century.

Healthy People 2010 identifies the leading health indicators intended to help everyone more easily understand the importance of health promotion and disease prevention and to encourage wide participation in improving health in the next decade.

Two of the 10 leading health indicators, (1) physical activity and (2) overweight and obesity, are the major focus of this book. Indicators affecting the health of people also include:

1. Physical activity
2. Overweight and obesity
3. Tobacco use
4. Substance abuse
5. Responsible sexual behavior
6. Mental health
7. Injury and violence
8. Environmental quality
9. Immunization
10. Access to health care

Physical Activity

Regular physical activity throughout life is important for maintaining a healthy body, enhancing psychological well-being, and preventing premature death. The evidence is growing and is more convincing than ever! People of all ages who are generally inactive can improve their health and well-being by becoming physically active. Despite the proven benefits of physical activity, more than 50% of American adults do not get enough physical activity to provide health benefits. Twenty-five percent of adults are not active at all in their leisure time.

Overweight and Obesity

These are major contributors to many preventable causes of death. On average, higher body weights are associated with high death rates.

In the United States, obesity has risen at an epidemic rate during the past 20 years. Research indicates that the situation is worsening rather than improving.

Where do we need to focus our efforts? The answer is in focusing on individuals changing their health-related lifestyles. That is why Chapter 1, about changing to a healthier lifestyle, forms the foundation of enhancing your health and wellness.

Fit to be Well: Essential Concepts offers simple, workable approaches for being healthy and fit that can easily be added into your lifestyle and schedule. A healthy lifestyle incorporates all facets of fitness. The goal is to introduce simple ways to integrate each of these elements into your daily life. As you progress through the chapters you will find easy-to-follow guidelines for:

- Modifying your lifestyle behaviors
- Increasing your self-esteem and creating a more positive self-image
- Eating a balanced and nutritional diet
- Keeping your body composition and weight at a healthy level
- Improving physical endurance, strength, and flexibility
- Managing stress

Fit to be Well aims to increase your awareness of each aspect of a physically fit lifestyle. By adding self-assessments and related labs to each of the chapters, this text becomes an interactive guide to building and implementing a fitness program that will work with your individual needs and schedule.

Getting Started

Right from the start, Chapter 1: Changing to a Healthy Lifestyle, has you actively participating as you learn how to effectively change your behavior. The nine chapters that follow provide a fitness road map that will guide you through:

- Preparing for Physical Activity and Exercise (Chapter 2),
- Improving Cardiorespiratory Endurance (Chapter 3),
- Increasing Flexibility (Chapter 4),
- Increasing Muscular Strength and Endurance (Chapter 5),
- Choosing a Nutritious Diet (Chapter 6),
- Maintaining a Healthy Body Composition and Body Weight (Chapter 7),
- Assessing Body Composition (Chapter 8)
- Managing Stress (Chapter 9), and
- Responsible Decision Making (Chapter 10).

You are the most important person taking care of your health. The key to taking responsibility for yourself is learning what works for you and then implementing what you have learned into your daily life. Some people view fitness-related goals as impossible dreams. The truth, however, is that everyone is capable of obtaining a healthy lifestyle. Keep in mind that every change you make is significant, no matter how big or small.

References

Myers J., Prakash M., Froelicher, V., Do D., Partington S., and Atwood, J. E. Exercise capacity and mortality among men referred for exercise testing. *New England Journal of Medicine*, March 14, 2002; 346:793–801.

Mokdad A., Marks J., Stroup D., and Gerberding J. Actual causes of death in the United States, 2000. *Journal of the American Medical Association*, March 10, 2004; 291:1238–1245.

U.S. Department of Health and Human Services (DHHS), Centers for Disease Control and Prevention (CDC). *Physical Activity and Health: A Report of the Surgeon General.* Atlanta, GA: DHHS, 1996. http://www.cdc.gov/nccdphp/sgr/sgr.htm.

U.S. DHHS. *Healthy People 2010: Understanding and Improving Health.* Washington, DC: DHHS, 2000. http://www.healthypeople.gov/

World Health Organization. Preamble to the Constitution of the World Health Organization as adopted by the International Health Conference, New York, 19–22 June, 1946; signed on 22 July 1946 by the representatives of 61 States (Official Records of the World Health Organization, no. 2, p. 100) and entered into force on 7 April 1948.

CHAPTER

1

Changing to a Healthy Lifestyle

Objectives

After reading this chapter, you should be able to:

- Describe the benefits of changing to a healthier lifestyle.
- Describe the Stages of Change model used in changing to a healthy lifestyle.
- Design a personal contract for changing a health-related behavior.

How Ready Are You to Change Your Behavior?

Determining Your Stage of Change

Everyone has a health behavior they would either like to adopt or an unhealthy behavior they would like to eliminate. Follow the steps below to see how ready you are for a health-related behavior change:

Step 1   **Identify a health behavior to change (write it on the line and be specific):**

_____

Step 2   **Find your current stage of change.**

Change Step 1's behavior into a question and write it on the line below. (For example: Do I get 7 to 9 hours of sleep most nights of the week? Do I consistently limit fat in my diet? Do I exercise for at least 30 minutes on most days of the week?)

_____

Step 3   **Read all of the possible answers to your question in Step 2 carefully. Circle the best response for your question.**

A. YES, I have been for MORE than 6 months.
B. YES, I have been, but for LESS than 6 months.
C. NO, but I intend to in the next 30 days.
D. NO, but I intend to in the next 6 months.
E. NO, and I do NOT intend to in the next 6 months.

Scoring

Answer choice (A)   Maintenance Stage
Answer choice (B)   Action Stage
Answer choice (C)   Preparation Stage
Answer choice (D)   Contemplation Stage
Answer choice (E)   Precontemplation Stage

Which stage are you in regarding the health-related behavior?

> **It is not the strongest of the species that survives,**
> **Nor the most intelligent,**
> **But the ones most responsive to change.**
>
> —Charles Darwin

Focus on Lifestyle

It is important to take a healthy look at your lifestyle. More than half of the leading causes of death in this country are preventable.

Actual causes of death are defined as lifestyle and behavioral factors, such as smoking and physical inactivity, that contribute to this nation's leading killers, including heart disease, cancer, and stroke (**Figure 1.1**). By changing these unhealthy behaviors people can improve their health and reduce their risk of disease.

Many individuals do not worry about their health until they lose it. Many have unsuccessfully tried various diets and a succession of exercise programs. This chapter offers methods, if used, that will enable you to develop a healthier lifestyle by changing a health-related behavior.

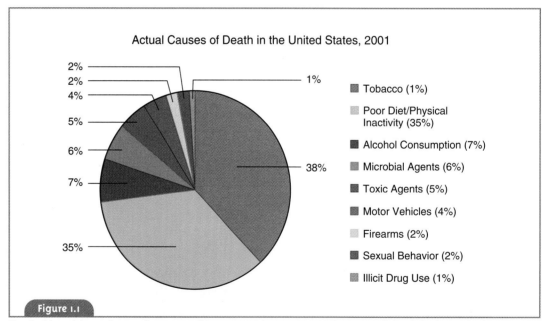

Actual Causes of Death in the United States, 2001

2%
2%
4%
5%
6%
7%
35%

1%
38%

- Tobacco (1%)
- Poor Diet/Physical Inactivity (35%)
- Alcohol Consumption (7%)
- Microbial Agents (6%)
- Toxic Agents (5%)
- Motor Vehicles (4%)
- Firearms (2%)
- Sexual Behavior (2%)
- Illicit Drug Use (1%)

Figure 1.1

Physical inactivity and poor diet are catching up to tobacco as actual causes of death in the United States. (*Source:* Modified from http://www.cdc.gov/nccdphp/factsheets/death_causes2000_access.htm.)

Changing Behavior

It is never very easy to change, and for some, it is extremely difficult. Why do some people find it so difficult to adhere to a healthy lifestyle and others find it easier? One answer involves the short-term pleasure of inappropriate behavior and the delayed nature of its negative health consequences. Some prefer dealing with life by playing the odds that they will not contract something like heart disease or cancer.

Research reveals that good educational programs can increase knowledge and foster positive attitudes. However, these factors have not been found to reliably influence long-term behavior change toward healthier lifestyles. While mastery of accurate information is necessary, it may not sufficiently empower most people with control of their behavior. On the other hand, the ability to use self-management techniques often helps individuals make lifestyle changes.

Prochaska and colleagues developed the Stages of Change model, which can help us to change a problem behavior (Prochaska, Norcross, and DiClemente 1994). This model says that people move through a series of stages of change (some call it a readiness to change). They describe behavior change as a process, not an event. Change does not happen overnight—it could take weeks, months, or even years.

In adopting healthy behaviors (e.g., regular physical activity) or eliminating unhealthy ones (e.g., eating saturated fat), people progress through five stages related to their readiness to change. At each stage, different intervention strategies help people progress to the next stage. The five distinct stages are:

1. Precontemplation
2. Contemplation
3. Preparation
4. Action
5. Maintenance

You can determine which stage of change you are presently in for any health behavior (starting or stopping a behavior) by using the simple questionnaire you completed in the Quick Start at the beginning of this chapter.

Progression through the stages of change is cyclical rather than linear. Rarely does a person successfully go through the stages sequentially without setbacks. Most people will recycle through the stages several times before being successful (Prochaska, Norcross, and DiClemente 1994). Figure 1.2 represents the stages of change in a graphical cyclic manner.

After identifying the stage of change you are in, the next step is to determine the appropriate processes of change to be used for the particular stage. These processes have also been referred to as techniques or strategies.

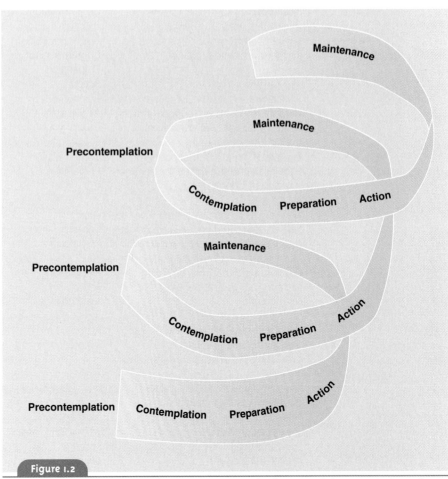

Figure 1.2

A spiral model of the stages of change. (*Source:* Prochaska J. O., DiClemente C. O., and Norcross J. C. In search of how people change: Applications to addictive behaviors. *American Psychologist 47*(1992): 1102–1114. Copyright ©1992 by the American Psychological Association. Reprinted by permission.)

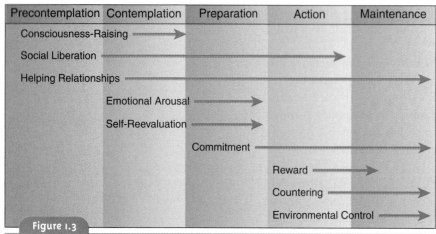

Figure 1.3

Select appropriate processes to promote change. (*Source:* Adapted from Prochaska J. O., Norcross J. C., and DiClemente C. O. *Changing for Good.* New York: Quill 2002. www.changecompanies.net/change_model.htm.)

Figure 1.3 matches the processes of changes and the stages of change.

Refer to **Table 1.1** for the major processes of change. These are activities and experiences that individuals engage in when they attempt to change a behavior.

The key to successful change is to determine what stage you are in, and then decide what processes (strategies) to use. There is no set time frame for each stage; you may spend more time in one stage than another. Change is a process that is unique to the individual and situation.

Table 1.1	Processes That Promote Change	
Processes of Change	**Stages of Change**	**Examples of Techniques**
Consciousness-raising: increased awareness	Precontemplation Contemplation	Read news stories or a book; watch a TV program; talk with a friend or doctor
Social liberation: societal support for the healthy behavior change	Precontemplation Contemplation Preparation Action	Availability of a health club; restaurants offering low-fat/low-carb foods
Helping relationships: support system of family, friends, and co-workers	All five stages	Discuss your plans with others; join with another who is working on the behavior
Emotional arousal: emotional experience related to the unhealthy behavior	Contemplation Preparation	Personal testimony of someone who has solved a similar behavioral problem; seeing someone suffering the harmful consequences of his or her unhealthy behavior
Self-reevaluation: understanding that your behavior is how you are known	Contemplation Preparation	See yourself as fit
Commitment: making a firm commitment to change and believing that it can be done	Preparation Action Maintenance	Make a New Year's resolution; tell others about your intentions
Reward: increasing the rewards for positive behavioral change and decreasing the rewards for unhealthy behavior	Action Maintenance	Reward the behavior change (e.g., buying new clothes, movie ticket)
Countering: substituting healthy behavior for an unhealthy behavior	Action Maintenance	Take a walk instead of watching TV
Environmental control: avoiding triggers or using cues	Action Maintenance	Avoid dessert parties; leave encouraging messages on a calendar or stuck to the mirror or refrigerator

Source: Adapted from Prochaska, J. O. Redding, C. A. and Evers, K. "The Transtheoretical Model and Stages of Change," in *Health Behavior and Health Education: Theory, Research, and Practice,* Glanz K., Lewis F. M., and Rimer B. K. (eds.), San Francisco: Jossey-Bass, 1996.

In addition to the stages and processes, the Stages of Change model features several other unique insights:

Weighing Pros and Cons

At each stage, a person weighs the pros and cons of adopting a new behavior. To help people move toward change, it is necessary to make the pros outweigh the cons. This is especially true in the precontemplation and contemplation stages.

Temptation

Change is difficult and a combination of cravings, emotional stress, and social situations can lead a person back to old habits. Should you slip or have a setback, do not think of this as a failure, but learn from it. What caused this setback? Now that you have learned this, avoid it next time!

Stage 1: Precontemplation

Precontemplation is the stage in which you are not ready to make a change in your life in the foreseeable future. Many individuals in this stage do not believe they have a problem and have often constructed defenses that aid in the denial of the problem. Many of us know that it is important to make healthy choices, but in a world full of temptations and unhealthy alternatives, it is often difficult to find the strength to make those changes in our lives.

Difficulty Living a Healthy Lifestyle

People often find it difficult to adhere to a healthy lifestyle of self-control because of:

- Firmly established habits
- Delayed gratification—people often want instant results or pleasure
- Delayed negative health consequences of an unhealthy lifestyle—it may take years or even decades before the effects are seen; "it won't happen to me" belief in which it is assumed that poor health happens to others but not me; prefer dealing with life by taking risks or playing the odds that they will not contract a disease or get injured
- Too much scientific information, which sometimes overwhelms or confuses
- Fear of failure—often based on past failed attempts
- Feeling a loss of control over one's life
- Too many choices from which to pick for type of exercise, food, and weight control

Stage 2: Contemplation

The contemplation stage occurs when you are aware that a problem exists and are seriously thinking about overcoming it, but have not yet made a commitment to take action. This is a time of reflection. Finding the reasons to change, the motivation to reach a goal, and the strength to make a plan work requires a lot of soul-searching. This stage can take a good amount of time and should not be rushed. As important as it is to make a healthy change in your life, take the time to find what truly motivates you and your behavior. This stage is the key to a successful course of action.

What Helps Change a Lifestyle?

Factors that influence an individual to change may include:

- Increasing knowledge can influence one's behavior, but often may not be enough to influence people to change. The maxim "Why do we do what we do, when we know what we know?" illustrates that knowledge often is insufficient to affect behavior.
- Motivation, having a reason—a person may want to change to avoid sickness, to look and feel better, to live longer, or because of pressure from a spouse, child, or friend.
- Readiness—motivation is required, but may involve physical capabilities as well. Another maxim—"You can lead a horse to water, but you can't make him drink"—may reflect a lack of motivation or perhaps the physical inability to act for a variety reasons.
- Landmark events—resolutions to change often occur at the start of a new year, on a birthday, upon the birth of a child, or the death of someone close to you.
- The ability to employ self-management techniques helps individuals to make lifestyle changes.

Motivation

Motivation is what drives us to make changes. No matter how big or how small the change may be, we must be inspired to make choices. Finding what inspires or motivates you is an essential step in making a successful adjustment in your lifestyle.

Motivations for change could include:

- Improving self-image and/or self-esteem
- Being a role model for someone else
- Improving relationships with family and peers
- Reducing stress
- Reducing risk of disease

Locus of Control

Life involves many struggles for control. Sometimes external factors can control aspects of your life for a moment. Other times the power is in your hands. The key to change is locating what controls a certain behavior. A locus of control is the figurative place where a person locates the source of responsibility in his or her life. It can be external or internal.

An external locus of control could be:

- Genetics
- Environmental factors—weather, location, etc.
- Another person or social group
- Other outside influences

An internal locus of control is:

- Self-expectations
- Internal thoughts ("I can do this")
- How open one is to change

In order to create a successful change in your life, you must be the one who takes the responsibility for your actions. Along with finding your motivation you need to find your locus of control.

Stage 3: Preparation

The preparation phase combines intention and behavior. Here you will monitor your behavior, analyze and identify patterns in your activity, and then set a goal. The most important concept in this stage is honesty. It is easy to try and make your behavior fit a certain pattern or profile. Sometimes the truth isn't what we want to see, but it is imperative in order to set realistic goals and to achieve real changes. Individuals are intending to take action within the next 30 days.

Self-Monitoring

Self-monitoring means observing and recording one's own behavior. This process is necessary to:

- Make you aware of the size and seriousness of a problem
- Provide a benchmark to compare your original behavior (point at which you began to try to change) with later behavior

Behaviors need recording as they occur, not days later. Self-monitoring devices to measure the frequency of a behavior include:

- Health notebook, journal, or diary to record the occurrence of a behavior
- Counters to collect data (e.g., pedometers, golf counters)
- Graph paper (horizontal axis represents time, usually days, and vertical axis represents the amount of the behavior to be changed—body weight, exercise, number of hours of sleep) (Table 1.2)

| Table 1.2 | Self-Managed Behavior Change Graph |

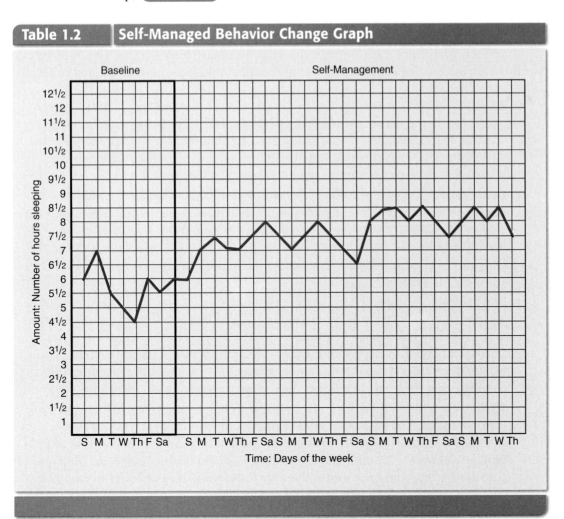

Analysis

Once you have gathered your data, sit back and review your record. You are looking for clues to why and how you engage in the unhealthy behavior you wish to change. You should look at the following:

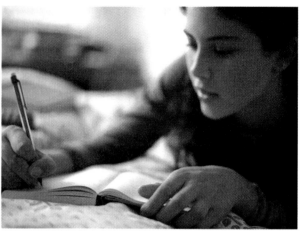

- **Time.** When during the day or week do you find yourself resorting to the activity? Is it linked with another activity (e.g., smoking after a meal or with a beer)?
- **Place.** Is there a specific place that you tend to be during the activity (e.g., making unhealthy diet choices on the way to class)?
- **Reason.** Can you link the behavior with a mood or an event that might trigger it (e.g., indulging in comfort food before an exam)?

Sometimes these aspects may not be immediately clear. Take a few days to look over your log. Remember, you are analyzing your behavior, not you as an individual. Keep a positive outlook—this behavior may be less than perfect, but you are making strides to change it, and that is more than the majority can say!

Goal Setting

You have determined the where, when, and why for your behavior in question. The next step is to set a goal. Don't rush through this step. You may think that the goal is obvious, but there are factors that must be taken into consideration in order for this goal to be effective. It must be:

- **Realistic.** While it is good to aim high, watch out for making your goal a bit too ambitious. If you make an unrealistic goal you will become frustrated along the way and lose your motivation quickly. Aim for a moderate expectation—one that will challenge you, but is within your ability. Remember you can always set a higher goal once you reach this one.
- **Quantitative.** Many times people set goals that are very abstract (i.e., wanting to lose weight). That is a fine ambition, but it is not an effective goal. You want your goal to be quantitative so that you can track your progress. A more effective goal would be to lose 10 pounds, or to stretch for 30 minutes three times a week. Try to define your goal in some type of measurable unit: minutes, pounds, number of servings, percentages, quantities, etc.
- **Broken down in steps.** If you start out thinking that you are aiming toward this one big goal from the beginning, you are going to find that it is easy to get discouraged during the first few weeks. You need to choose a goal that can be broken down into smaller intermediate steps—mini goals—along the way. For example, if the goal is to stop drinking soda, perhaps the mini goals could be to cut back to three sodas a day, then two, then one, and so on. Make sure your mini goals are quantitative.
- **Tracked on a timeline.** Having the ambition to live a healthy lifestyle is different than your goal. The ambition can be carried with you for as long as you want. The goal, however, must have an end date. By using a timeline it is easier to keep your progress on track. The end date is not the end of the healthy behavior. After you have completed your goal within the time frame you chose, be sure to continue practicing the healthy habits until they stick!

■ **Important to you.** If you do not feel that this goal is important or worthwhile, it will not be a success. It does not matter how many people tell you that your goal is great, you have to believe in it yourself. If you don't, go back and revise the goal until it fits with your expectations and your motivation.

Stage 4: Action

The action stage is where you begin to move toward a healthier behavior. You have your motivation, your internal locus of control, and your goal. You are ready to make this change! Having a plan and a contract will help further your success as you begin to reach toward your goal. See a personal contract in Figure 1.4 . Action involves the most observable behavioral changes and requires considerable commitments of time and energy.

PERSONAL CONTRACT

Start Date: _____ Finish Date: _____

The Goal: _____

Motivation (benefits): _____

Identify your current stage of change (see Quick Start, page 1): _____

Match your current stage of change and other stages you anticipate progressing through with the appropriate processes of change (see Figure 1.3):

_____   _____

_____   _____

What specific techniques will you use for each of the processes identified above (see Table 1.1)?	
Processes	Specific techniques
Stage of change on the finish date:	

I, _____, agree to work toward a healthier lifestyle and in doing so shall comply with the terms and dates of this contract.

Signature: _____ Date: _____

Witness: _____ Date: _____

Figure 1.4

A personal contract to bind yourself to your chosen course of action.

1

Tipping Point

Rewards

- Self-contracting means you establish and administer your own rewards.
- Rewards are meant as motivation to keep the momentum going until you reach your goal.
- Rewards should be given immediately and frequently but in moderate amounts.
- Tailor your rewards to your individual taste—make sure they are desirable enough to motivate you.
- The reward should not be associated with the negative behavior you are trying to change. For example, if you are trying to lose weight, don't make your reward a brownie.

The Plan

The plan is where you break your goal down into manageable steps. Your plan should include:

- What you will need. Do you need a newly stocked cabinet with healthier food? Do you need a gym membership? What equipment will you need for each of your steps?
- What is your timeline? When will you start this plan? When is your ending date for your goal?
- The steps you will take. Your goal should be broken down into smaller mini goals, each with their own timeline.

The Contract

Write a contract binding yourself to the chosen course of action. Your contract should include:

- **Start Date** Write the date that you will begin your plan.
- **Finish Date** Write the date when you will have completed your goal.
- **The Goal** Be specific and concise.
- **Motivation (benefits)** Determine what is in it for you.
- **Identify your current stage of change** See Quick Start.
- **Identify the processes (strategies) of change** Use Figure 1.3 for each possible stage of change.
- **For each process of change to be used, identify a specific technique.** See Table 1.1.
- **Identify the stage of change when you finish.** See Quick Start.
- **Your signature** Sign your name as a sign of your commitment to your plan.
- **Witness signature** Have a close friend or family member sign your contract as well.

Tipping Point

Contracting with Others

- Contracting with another person makes the contract a public commitment.
- This person should have a meaningful relationship with you—a roommate, friend, parent, or relative, for example.
- Have this person review your contract and sign it as a witness to your new commitment.
- A commitment to friends and family is less likely to be broken than just a personal commitment.

The Inside Track

Graduated Regimen Implementation

Starting a new behavior or stopping a behavior all at once is difficult.

Graduated programs can shape desired behaviors. Example: slowly start exercising.

Stage 5: Maintenance

After at least 6 months in the action stage, the person may move into the fifth stage: maintenance. This phase is when you keep up the new healthier habits that have replaced the old habits. Change is maintained more easily now. There may be an initial excitement associated with making a change in which your motivation and commitment will both be high and the outlook toward your goal is positive. But sometimes this phase can dwindle down, leaving the success of your plan vulnerable to barriers.

The five main barriers to successful change are:

- Social impact
- Stress
- Postponing
- Justification
- Denying rsesponsibility

Social Impact

There can be both positive and negative social impacts on your plan to change a behavior.

Positive social impacts may be in the form of:

- Structured support groups
- Cheerleading by friends and family
- Role models—people around you to whom you look up to and admire

Negative social impacts may include:

- Feeling like the odd one out
- Peer pressure
- Attending functions that tempt you to break your contract

Tipping Point

Dealing with Negative Social Impact

- Realize that this is your individual goal. Not everyone around you will have the same intentions as you.
- Stay committed to your goal. Review your contract before you go out to remind yourself how important this change is to you.
- Try and choose healthy alternatives whenever possible.
- Be a role model to others. By sticking with your plan and committing yourself to a healthier lifestyle, you may motivate others to do the same!
- Have a friend who wants you to push the limits of your goal? Assign that person as your personal coach or cheerleader. By making them feel like a responsible party in your plan, they may very well take on a role of support rather than peer pressure!

Let those around you know that you are trying to change this specific behavior. They may be able to offer tips and suggestions to help you along. More importantly, by explaining your goals to them they are more likely to respect your decision and less likely to pressure you into relapsing into old behavior patterns.

Stress

What's the word...

stress The physical and emotional tension that comes from situations the body perceives as threatening.

procrastination Pushing a task to a later point in time.

rationalization Making excuses for not carrying out a task.

blaming Placing the responsibility of an unmet goal on someone else.

One of the biggest barriers to changing lifestyle behaviors is **stress**. Stress can occur anywhere in our daily lives and without the correct management techniques it can lead you away from your goal. Eating comfort food, drinking, and other reckless behavior are common ways that many people deal with stress—none of which are effective or healthy. Learning effective coping techniques can not only make it easier for you to stay on track with your plan of action, but will help you to create a better sense of wellness overall.

When life throws curve balls at you try these helpful tips to calm down and get back on track:

- Close your eyes and count to ten. Take deep breaths between each number.
- Have a CD on hand with calming music. Put it on and focus on the music for 5 minutes.
- Keep a journal. Record how you feel; sometimes just getting your thoughts on paper can help release tension.
- Go for a short brisk walk. The change of scenery and fresh air can renew your mood.
- Stop, stretch your muscles, and breathe deeply.

Postponement

After that initial surge of motivation in the beginning of the action phase, it can get difficult to muster the energy to continue to make the healthy choices. Many times the steps to reaching your goal get pushed aside, postponed until a later point in time. It is best to stop the procrastination as soon as you feel yourself slipping into that mindset.

When you realize that you are postponing a step in your plan:

- Stop and identify out loud that you are procrastinating.
- Try and pin down why you are avoiding that particular step. For example, is the cold weather causing you to avoid going to the gym? Or is that healthy dish too time-consuming to make?
- Once you have identified why you are postponing a particular step, try to revise that step to fit better with your life. For example, buy a few exercise videos for working out at home when the weather is bad. Or, find simpler recipes that still offer the same nutritional value.

Tipping Point

Avoiding Procrastination

- Mark your calendar, daily planner, or appointment book.
- Leave messages on the refrigerator, bulletin board, wall calendar, next to the bed, or on the bathroom mirror.
- Set your alarm, enter your goal in your computer, or have a friend call you.

Justification

Many times when we procrastinate we justify or **rationalize** our actions. We make excuses for why we have not completed the task. It is important to catch yourself if you find that you are justifying not meeting your goal or one of your steps. Your plan may quickly become a slippery slope where nothing is accomplished, but everything is rationalized. When you feel your self making excuses:

- Say your excuse out loud and listen—is it credible?
- Write down those times when you push your task off and why you did so. If you find yourself falling off course with your goal, these logs will provide a good resource to when and why you aren't meeting each step.
- Understand that there will be times when you can't complete a step that second. Make sure that you are justifying the valid procrastinations, not the ones made out of low motivation.

Denying Responsibility

Along with justification can come **blaming**. Blaming is where you displace the responsibility for missing a step or not completing a goal onto someone else. Because of *him/her/them* or what *they* did, the goal was not met. This is an easy trap to fall into as it is convenient and gives the appearance that you are not at fault. You are the victim. No matter how good blaming looks on paper, it will not help you reach your goal. You will still be left with an unfinished plan. It is important to accept responsibility for your own actions.

Relapse

Relapse can occur at any stage of the change process. It can be triggered by many things: an extra stressful day or week, an unexpected event, low levels of motivation, etc. If you find yourself relapsing along the way try to identify a reason. Are you losing motivation? Is your plan unrealistic? Do you not have the right equipment or facilities?

This is a process; nothing is set in stone. You have the freedom to go back and revise your goal at any time. Don't be afraid to reevaluate your plan. If something is not working for you, find alternatives that will still help you change the behavior. Most importantly: Do not give up! A relapse is normal, it doesn't mean that you are not able to complete your goals. It is a minor setback that can be overcome.

Acceptance

Acceptance is the finish line. The old unhealthy behavior has been fully replaced at this point. Not only have you completed your goal, but you have integrated healthy habits into your daily routine. Be aware that this stage may not come quickly. Achieving your goal and dealing with relapses may take a long while, but your healthy new lifestyle is definitely worth it.

Conclusion

Lifestyle change is a process that involves many steps and a lot of persistence. It is possible to have multiple changes taking place at once. The chapters in this text provide a wealth of information on many different aspects of healthy living. By incorporating each topic into your daily life, you will be working toward a more rounded sense of wellness.

Reflect >>>> Reinforce >>>> Reinvigorate

Knowledge Check

Answers in Appendix D

1. What is the first stage of change?
   - A. Preparation
   - B. Precontemplation
   - C. Action
2. An effective plan for changing a behavior should have:
   - A. The steps to be taken
   - B. How long it will last
   - C. List of items needed
   - D. All of the above
3. Which factors influence a person to change?
   - A. Obtaining more knowledge
   - B. The ability to use self-management skills
   - C. Having a reason
   - D. All of the above

Modern Modifications

The chapters in this text illustrate a wide variety of the important aspects of a healthy lifestyle. In each chapter there will be a section in which you will be given a chance to:

- Take a moment to look at your lifestyle in the terms of topic discussed. What would you like to change in that area of your life?
- Go through and pick one of the suggestions provided. These suggestions are meant to be easily absorbed into your daily routine and offer immediate opportunities for change.
- Congratulate yourself. You are one step closer to a happier healthier lifestyle. Even small changes can make a big difference!

Critical Thinking

Answers in Appendix D

Scenario One: Angela is trying to improve her performance in ballet. Which of the following would be the best goal for her:

A. Improve flexibility

B. Dance more artistically

C. Stretch at least 30 minutes a day

Scenario Two: Max is thinking about making a change in his life. He is brainstorming about what motivates him and is trying to identify where his locus of control is. Which stage of change is Max in currently?

A. Action

B. Relapse

C. Contemplation

Scenario Three: John is upset that he didn't complete one of the steps to his goal. He is claiming that Debbie's actions prevented him from achieving that particular step. What barrier has John encountered?

A. Stress

B. Blaming

C. Justification

D. All of the above

Going Above and Beyond

Websites

MedlinePlus: Exercise and Physical Fitness
http://www.nlm.nih.gov/medlineplus/exercisephysicalfitness.html

Physician and Sports Medicine
http://www.physsportsmed.com

Morbidity and Mortality Weekly Report
http://www.cdc.mmwr.gov

Transtheoretical Model
www.uri.edu/research/cprc/transtheoretical.htm

References and Suggested Readings

DHHS. *Healthy People 2010*. Washington, DC: DHHS, 2000.

DHHS. *Physical Activity and Health: A Report of the Surgeon General*. Atlanta, GA: DHHS, 1996.

Marcus B., et al., Assessing motivational readiness and decision-making for exercise. *Health Psychology* 22(1992): 257–261.

Prochaska J. O. Strong and weak principles for progressing from precontemplation to action on the basis of twelve problem behaviors. *Health Psychology* 13(1994): 47–51.

Prochaska J. O. and Markus B. H. "The Transtheoretical Model: Applications to Exercise," in *Advances in Exercise Adherence*, Dishman, R. K. (ed.), Champaign, IL: Human Kinetics, 1994.

Prochaska J. O. and Velicer W. F. The transtheoretical model of health behavior change, *American Journal of Health Promotion* 12(1)(1997): 38–48.

Prochaska J. O., Norcross J. C., and DiClemente C. O. *Changing for Good*. New York: HarperCollins Publishers, 1994. Reprinted by Quill, 2002.

Zimmerman G. L. et al. "A 'Stages of Change' Approach to Helping Patients Change Behavior." *American Family Physician*, March 1, 2000: American Academy of Family Physicians.

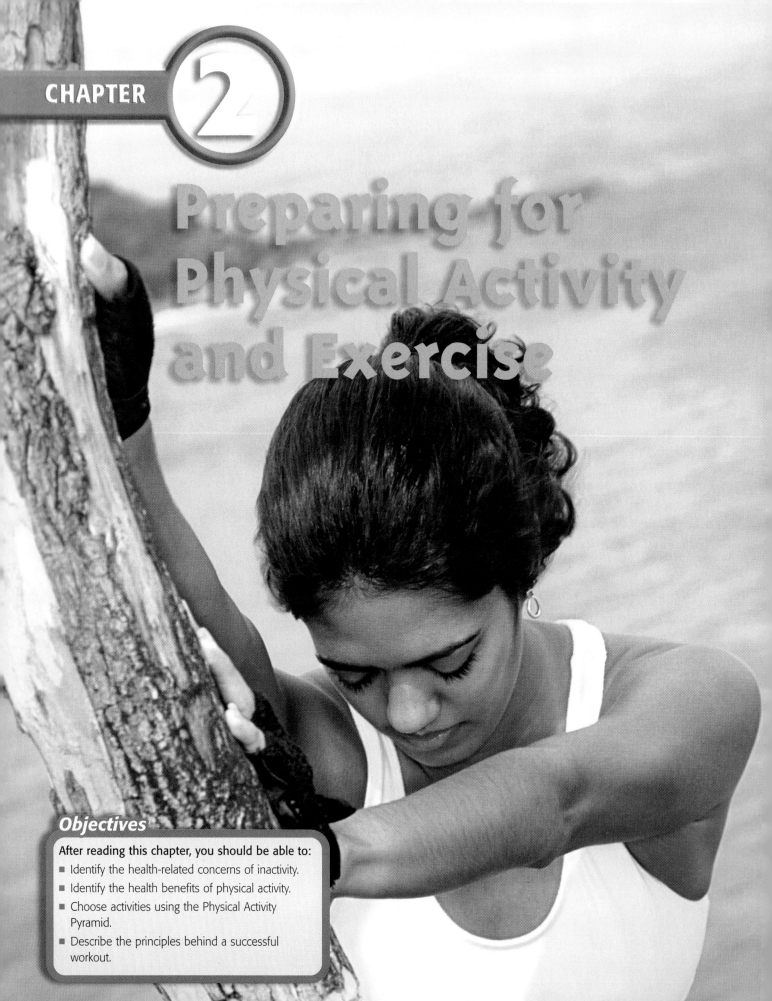

CHAPTER 2

Preparing for Physical Activity and Exercise

Objectives

After reading this chapter, you should be able to:

- Identify the health-related concerns of inactivity.
- Identify the health benefits of physical activity.
- Choose activities using the Physical Activity Pyramid.
- Describe the principles behind a successful workout.

A Walk to Health

What Do I Need to Begin?

- Loose, comfortable clothes
- Walking or cross-training shoes—preferably in good condition
- Hat
- Sunscreen
- Bottle of water
- A safe place to walk
- Time—will vary depending on the speed and distance you walk and an adequate amount of time to warm up and cool down

What Benefits Will I Receive?

- Increases self-esteem and positive self-image
- Reduces risk of certain diseases
- Builds strong bones
- Helps achieve and maintain a healthy weight
- Reduces stress
- Provides time for personal reflection
- Increases your time outdoors
- Provides quality time alone or with family/friends

How Do I Prepare for a Brisk Walk?

- **Rest.** Get an adequate amount of sleep the night before.
- **Hydrate.** You should be drinking 17–20 ounces of water 2–3 hours before the walk. Drink another 7–10 ounces 10–20 minutes before you step off. Continue to hydrate as you walk (Pfeiffer and Mangus 2004).
- **Warm up.** Walk around for 5 to 10 minutes while swinging your arms. This will get your circulation going.
- **Stretch.** After you warm up take the time to stretch the major muscle groups (quadriceps, hamstrings, calves, etc.) that you will be using. See Chapter 4 for detailed instructions on how to perform these and other important stretches.

How Should I Begin My Walk?

- Start off with a half-mile and gradually work your way up to two miles.
- Walk at your own comfort level, increasing the speed and distance only when you feel ready.
- Always wear sunscreen and a hat when walking outdoors—even in the winter!
- Remember to hydrate before, during, and after your walk.
- Cool down after you walk. Reduce your speed and continue walking slowly for 5 minutes. Stretch the major muscle groups again.
- Conclude this activity by taking a few deep breaths and relaxing.

2

Recent Trends of Inactivity and Health-Related Concerns

Daily activity may affect health more than any other factor—more than physical environment, even more than genetics. Diseases and disabilities are often not inevitable consequences of the aging process.

Dangers of Inactivity

Millions of Americans suffer from chronic illnesses that can be prevented or improved through regular physical activity. Inactivity can contribute to and/or exacerbate each of the following conditions that relate to the leading causes of death **Figure 2.1**:

- Coronary heart disease
- Heart attacks
- Diabetes
- Colon cancer
- Bone fractures
- High blood pressure
- Obesity

Who Is Active?

Less than 50% of adults achieve the recommended amount of regular physical activity **Figure 2.2**. In fact, 16% of all adults are not active at all (NCCDPHP 2001).

As part of the National Health Survey, The National Center for Health Statistics interviewed over 68,000 adults age 18 and older and found the following:

- Three out of 10 adults were physically active on a regular basis.

Figure 2.1

Leading causes of death in the United States, 2001. (*Source:* National Center for Health Statistics (NCHS) Vital Statistics System. *10 Leading Causes of Deaths, United States,* 2002. www.cdc.gov/ncipc/.)

Bar chart — Percent of All Deaths:

- Heart disease: 28.5
- Cancer: 22.8
- Stroke: 6.7
- Chronic lower respiratory disease: 5.1
- Unintentional injuries: 4.4
- Diabetes: 3
- Influenza and pneumonia: 2.7
- Alzheimer's disease: 2.4
- Kidney disease: 1.7
- Blood infection: 1.4
- All others: 21.4

Figure 2.2

Pie chart:
- 45% — Achieved the recommended amount of physical activity
- 39% — Were insufficient in the amount of physical activity
- 16% — Were inactive

Physical activity statistics in the United States, 2001. (*Source:* National Center for Chronic Disease Prevention and Health Promotion (NCCDPHP). "U.S. Physical Activity Statistics: 2001 State Summary Data," 2001.)

- Young white males were most likely to exercise.
- Nearly 8 out of 10 adults with graduate-level degrees engaged in some form of leisure-time physical activity, which was twice as many as those with less than a high school diploma.
- Adults with incomes of at least four times the poverty level were twice as likely to engage in regular leisure-time physical activity than adults with incomes below the poverty line.
- Married men and women were most likely to be physically active.
- Single adults who had never been married were most likely to engage in strengthening activities such as weight lifting.
- Widowed adults were less likely than married adults to engage in physical activities.
- 67% of adults living in the western United States were physically active, compared to 56% of those living in the South.
- Adults living in the suburbs were more likely to be physically active than those in urban or rural areas.
- Nearly half of young adults aged 12–21 are not vigorously active on a regular basis.

Benefits of Physical Activity

Physical activity is a huge component of wellness. A common misconception is that increasing your activity level only helps your physical health. This couldn't be more wrong. The benefits of physical activity involve all aspects of wellness, which combine to create an improved sense of well-being.

According to the National Center for Chronic Disease Prevention and Health Promotion, "people who enjoy participating in moderate intensity or vigorous intensity physical activity on a regular basis benefit by lowering their risk of developing coronary heart disease, stroke, non-insulin-dependent (type 2) diabetes mellitus, high blood pressure, and colon cancer by 30–50%." In addition, physical activity "reduces feelings of depression and anxiety, promotes psychological well-being and reduces feelings of stress" (NCCDPHP 2004).

Exercise is a great way to relieve stress. It reduces muscle tension; stimulates regular, deep breathing; increases blood levels of endorphins; and creates an opportunity to free the mind from worries. The next time you exercise, see if you can become aware of these four stages of stress relief through exercise:

Stage 1: Paying Attention

At the beginning of an exercise session, focus your mind on the activity and allow any thoughts that arise to pass out of your mind. When you notice them, simply say to yourself, "Oh, I have a thought," and bring yourself back to focusing on your activity.

Stage 2: Interested Attention

After a period of concentrating and letting go, you no longer have to concentrate on eliminating distractions, and you sense a flowing with the activity.

Stage 3: Absorbed Attention

Absorption with the activity is so great that it is very difficult for you to be distracted by what is going on around you. You may experience altered perceptions of space and time, and your mind may move through thoughts and images without your direction. The experience can be dream-like, except you are entirely awake and attentive.

Stage 4: Merging

You no longer are aware of any separation between you and what you are doing. The experience of union is complete: physical, mental, and spiritual. You attain a complete loss of self-consciousness, and even though you may be working your body very hard, mentally and spiritually you feel very calm.

Figure 2.3

Stages of exercise-induced relaxed concentration. (*Source:* Edlin G et al. *Health and Wellness, 7th Edition.* Sudbury, MA: Jones and Bartlett, 2002:142.)

Check Your Health Status Before Starting

Moderate physical activity programs are not dangerous for most people, and no medical clearance is needed.

Complete the Physical Activity Readiness Questionnaire (PAR-Q) (Lab 2.1). If you answered "yes" to any of the checklist items, discuss your answers with a physician *before* having your fitness assessed or starting a fitness program.

The American Heart Association suggests that you see a doctor before exercising if:

- You have a heart condition
- You take medicine for your heart and/or blood pressure
- You get pains in your chest, left side of your neck, or your left shoulder or arm when you exercise
- Your chest has been hurting for about a month
- You tend to get dizzy, lose consciousness, and fall
- Mild exertion leaves you breathless
- You have bone or joint problems that a doctor told you could be worsened by exercise
- You have an overweight or obesity problem
- Have a medical condition, such as insulin-dependent diabetes, that requires special attention in an exercise program
- You are middle-aged or older (40 years for men; 50 years for women)

Become Familiar with the Components of Physical Fitness

It is easy to become confused regarding the terms of physical activity and exercise. In this context, physical activity is any activity that engages the body, while exercise is considered a series of coordinated movements specifically intended to increase physical performance. Both physical activity and exercise are essential when creating a balanced workout.

Physical Activity

Physical activity includes any activity that gets you up and moving throughout the day. These activities could include grocery shopping, mowing the lawn, taking the dog for a walk, shoveling a driveway, etc. While they may not be specifically intended to increase your muscular or cardiovascular endurance, daily physical activities are just as important as structured exercise.

Exercise

There are four different elements of exercise that provide the basis of a balanced workout program. Remember, these components are made up of structured activities aimed at increasing specific elements of fitness. The Centers for Disease Control and Prevention (CDC) define these "components of physical fitness" as:

- **Cardiorespiratory endurance:** "the ability of the body's circulatory and respiratory systems to supply fuel during sustained physical activity."
- **Muscle strength and endurance:** "the ability of the muscle to exert force during an activity . . . and . . . the ability of the muscle to continue to perform without fatigue."
- **Flexibility:** "the range of motion around a joint."
- **Body composition:** "the relative amount of muscle, fat, bone, and other vital parts of the body."

The Physical Activity Pyramid

The Physical Activity Pyramid **Figure 2.4** promotes a balanced diet of weekly physical activity. It suggests a healthy dose of daily physical activity combined with certain amounts of the four components of exercise. The pyramid follows the Frequency, Intensity, Time, and Type (FITT) guidelines with each level outlining the:

Figure 2.4

The exercise and physical activity pyramid. (*Source:* The Activity Pyramid © 2003 Park Nicollet Health Innovations, Minneapolis, U.S.A. 1-888-637-2675. Reprinted with permission.)

2

Frequency of the activity: The number of times an exercise or group of exercises is performed within a certain time frame. Usually this is measured in sessions per week. How frequently you perform a certain exercise depends on the intensity of the exercise.

Intensity of the activity: The amount of energy exerted while performing an exercise.

Time or duration of the activity: The measurement of how long an exercise or group of exercises takes to complete.

Type of activity: The classification of exercise. Daily activity, cardiorespiratory endurance, muscle strength, and flexibility are all different types of activities.

Cumulative Moderate Activity

It can be difficult to try and set aside large blocks of time each day for exercise when you are first beginning a fitness regimen. The great news about daily physical activity (Level 1 on the pyramid) is that you can accumulate a moderate amount of activity throughout the week. A moderate amount of physical activity is roughly equivalent to physical activity that uses approximately 150 calories of energy per day, or 1000 calories per week. This can be achieved in a variety of ways. (**Table 2.1**) illustrates the number of calories burned per minute for a variety of daily activities. If you only have a couple of short intervals of time to work out each week, you would choose a more intense exercise. Or, if you have large frequent blocks of time, a less vigorous exercise may be more appropriate.

Table 2.1	Calories Used by Everyday Activities*	
	Calories Used in 10 Minutes[†]	
Activities	Women	Men
Walking fast	45	60
Painting	45	60
Weeding	45	60
Washing a car	45	60
Playing tag with a child	50	67
Mowing the lawn	55	73
Square dancing	55	73
Scrubbing floors	55	73
Hiking off-trail	60	80
Biking to work	60	80
Shoveling snow	60	80
Moving furniture	60	80
Walking upstairs	70	93
Cross-country skiing	80	106
Backpacking	80	106
Running upstairs	150	200

*Use an average of 200 calories a day by doing these activities and decrease your risk of disease and live longer, without ever going near a gym or treadmill.

[†]Figures are for a 132-pound woman and a 176-pound man. All values are approximate and will vary from person to person.

Source: Edlin, G. and Golanty, E. *Health and Wellness, 8th Edition.* Sudbury, MA: Jones and Bartlett, 2004:133.

For every physical activity or exercise session be sure to **warm up** before and **cool down** after. Skipping over or rushing through these two phases of an activity can be dangerous.

The Warm-up

- Takes 5 to 10 minutes of low-intensity movement, such as walking, before stretching inactive muscles.
- Prepares your body for physical activity by gradually increasing muscle temperature and metabolism.
- Increases blood flow and oxygen delivery to the muscles, protects tendons, and lengthens short, tight muscles.
- Gives the body a chance to redirect blood to active muscles.
- Gives the heart time to adapt to increased demands.
- Ends with stretching the major joints with some range-of-motion movements.

The Cool-down

- Takes 5 to 10 minutes using the same muscles just exercised at a reduced pace.
- Consists of light, general movements and stretching or ending your chosen physical activity gradually.
- Helps to avoid the pooling of blood in the muscles and to remove metabolic end-products such as lactic acid and carbon dioxide.
- Determines how you feel several hours after your activity, as it can reduce muscle soreness, cramps, and stiffness.
- Ending with stretching also improves flexibility. Some experts feel it is best done at the end of the cool-down rather than while warming up.

What's the word. . .

warm-up The 5–10 minutes of low-intensity movement at the beginning of a workout that prepares the body for activity by increasing muscle temperature and metabolism.

cool-down The 5–10 minutes at the end of a workout involving light movement and stretching.

overload Placing a greater-than-normal amount of stress (within reason) on the body in order to make it function at a higher capacity.

specificity The type of physical changes you desire in your body relates directly to the type of exercise you choose.

progression The gradual increase of the level and intensity of exercise.

The Principles of a Successful Workout

Physical fitness is dependent on many different factors. The following principles should be taken into account when designing an exercise program:

Overload.   In order for an exercise to have an effect on the body, there has to be some level of stress placed on it. Overload refers to placing a greater-than-normal amount of stress (within reason) on the body in order to make it function at a higher capacity, therefore, increasing endurance and/or strength.

Specificity.   The type of physical changes you desire in your body relates directly to the type of exercise you choose.

Progression.   By gradually increasing the frequency, intensity, and duration of exercise, the body is able to gain improvement in strength and endurance.

Reversibility. The results of physical fitness are not permanent. If you become inactive for an extended period of time, you may lose a good portion of strength and endurance that you have built up. It is important to maintain your fitness level with regular activity.

Consistency. The only way to keep in shape is to participate in physical activities on a frequent and regular basis. Sporadic bouts of exercise will not result in increased fitness levels.

Individual differences. We all differ in the maximum level of fitness we can and want to achieve. What works for one may not work as well for another.

Safety. Train, don't strain. Safety involves being aware of all aspects of your exercise routine. From the correct way to use a machine to knowing the limits of your body, there are numerous things that you should pay attention to in order to keep your body safe and healthy while you exercise.

Rest. Your body needs rest to recover from strenuous workouts. Back-to-back high-intensity workouts only break down muscles, and never give them a chance to grow stronger.

Tipping Point

Tips for Workouts

- Hard workout days should be followed by easy workout days or rest.
- Alternate between lifting weights and aerobic exercise from day to day.
- High-energy days should be your harder workout days.
- On low-energy days simply rest or perform a light workout.
- Most of all: Listen to your body!

Stay Motivated

Selecting an exercise that is right for you is only the first step in a successful exercise program. Making the necessary adjustments in your life to accommodate this new lifestyle change can be difficult. Procrastination, social pressures, stress, and busy schedules can hinder progress. Here are proven strategies to help motivate you to start exercising and to stay with it:

- Develop an exercise habit. Keep at it, knowing the more consistent you are in the beginning, the more fixed your new activity will become.
- Reserve a time slot each day for working out, and don't let anything interfere.
- Don't let others lead you astray. Inform everyone of your exercise time and that you would appreciate them respecting your choice.
- Seek support from friends and family, and believe that you can succeed.
- Be patient with yourself. Some days you will be more motivated or have more time than other days. A brief period of not exercising is not a disaster.
- Plan ahead and follow your plan. Decide when, where, how often, and with whom you will work out. Be prepared to exercise.
- Team up. Exercising with others can motivate you when you'd rather not exercise. But it can have a down side. A less motivated or less optimistic partner, for example, can drain you.
- Set realistic exercise goals. Set goals that you not only know you can achieve, but that are specific, not vague.

- Keep an exercise record. Attach an **exercise log** to your refrigerator, in your bedroom, or office and record each session.
- Have fun. Customize your approach to make exercise more enjoyable. For instance, read, watch television, or listen to your favorite music while pedaling a stationary cycle.
- Add variety. Select activities that you enjoy. **Cross-training** helps.
- Affirm your efforts out loud each morning.
- Listen to your body. Your body may need a break at times.
- Complement exercise. In addition to exercising, be sure to eat a low-fat, balanced diet, sleep well, and avoid unhealthy influences like smoking and high stress.

For Exercise Drop-outs: How to Get Started Again

More than half the people who enroll in supervised exercise programs drop out within the first 6 months. So chances are, if you start exercising, at some point you are going to stop. Despite your best intentions, vacations, illnesses, and work responsibilities may wreak havoc on your regimen. How can you keep little breaks in your exercise program from meaning that you will never again break a sweat?

- Stop beating yourself up. Remind yourself that it is just a temporary suspension of your program. Look upon every relapse as a learning experience.
- Reevaluate your goals. Are you going to plan to stay on a 2-hour-a-day program 365 days a year for 10 years? If so, you're setting yourself up to fail. Instead, set realistic goals with more activity some days and less on others.
- Get going. Perform some kind of physical activity today.
- Continually plan. If you are planning a trip or your workload picks up, think of strategies for incorporating short periods of physical activity into your day, which may prevent relapse.
- Most people find themselves starting over again at some point in time after dropping out of an exercise program. It is difficult to determine the long-term impact of a start-stop-start-stop pattern of exercise on health, although there may be a cumulative beneficial effect.

> **What's the word...**
>
> **exercise log** A record of your activity that includes the type, duration, and intensity of each exercise each day.
>
> **cross-training** Combining the components of fitness in a workout program, instead of focusing on only one area.

Stay Safe

Physical activity comes with safety risks. Learning how to protect your body from injury and illness can make your fitness program that much more enjoyable. Here are some general guidelines for staying safe while staying active:

- Do not exercise if you have a cold or flu, and never exercise if you have a fever, chest pain, or breathing problem.
- Drink plenty of water. Do not wait until you are thirsty to drink water. You should be drinking 7–10 ounces of water for every 10–20 minutes of activity (Pfeiffer 2004).

- Do not exercise if you have not had enough sleep, are fasting, or have just eaten. Save your meals for after exercise, and wait at least 2 hours after a heavy meal before exercising.
- Factors that can negatively affect your ability to handle extreme temperatures include: not dressing appropriately for conditions, inadequate nutrition, dehydration, alcohol consumption, certain medications, and health conditions such as diabetes and heart disease.
- Wear the proper clothing, shoes, and equipment to prevent injuries.

Be the Best and Expect the Best

Physical activity is essential to healthy living. It can ward off disease, relieve stress, and help increase self-esteem. By subscribing to a balanced diet of exercise and accumulating a moderate amount of daily physical activity, you are well on your way to a life of wellness. The following chapters in this book are designed to give you a gradual learning experience in fitness. The upcoming material will answer your questions, help you increase your understanding of physical activity, and achieve a healthy lifestyle.

Tipping Point

Dress properly by following the guidelines below:
- Wear clothing specific to the activity.
- Clothes should be comfortable and allow you to move freely.
- Cotton or cotton/polyester blend is recommended to allow for sweat evaporation.
- DO NOT wear clothing that restricts sweat evaporation. Sweating is how the body regulates its internal temperature.
- Wear additional clothing in layers to warm up or cool down as needed.
- The best protection against wind and rain is an outer layer that allows heat loss and sweat evaporation (e.g., Gortex).
- Women should consider wearing an exercise bra, and men, sports underwear (e.g., compression shorts or jockstrap).
- Protective equipment is needed for some activities (e.g., helmet for bikers and inline skating).

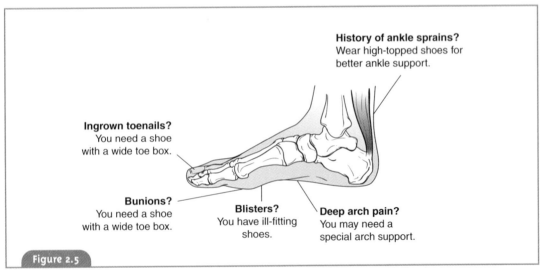

History of ankle sprains?
Wear high-topped shoes for better ankle support.

Ingrown toenails?
You need a shoe with a wide toe box.

Bunions?
You need a shoe with a wide toe box.

Blisters?
You have ill-fitting shoes.

Deep arch pain?
You may need a special arch support.

Figure 2.5

Foot problems may be related to your footwear.

Tipping Point

The American Orthopedic Foot and Ankle Society makes several recommendations for selecting a good fitting shoe (**Figure 2.5** and **Figure 2.6**):

- Have both feet measured when they are at their largest: at the end of the day or after a run, walk, game, or practice.
- Wear your workout socks.
- Try on the shoes, because sizes vary by manufacturer.
- Make sure both shoes fit.
- Ensure that the shoe provides at least one thumb's width of space from the longest toe to the end of the toe box.

A variety of athletic shoes exist: running/jogging, walking, tennis, court, and cross-training. Properly sized socks help prevent blisters, ingrown toenails, and absorb perspiration.

Athletic shoes should have:

Ankle collar padding—for fit and comfort; notched area to reduce pressure on Achilles tendon

Support—to stabilize the heel and support arch (some activities may need high-top shoe)

Tongue—well padded to prevent irritation

Space—enough room to wiggle toes

Cushioning—heel and midsole

Figure 2.6

Carefully select your athletic footwear.

The Inside Track

If you start to notice pain in your feet, ankles, legs, or knees though you haven't changed your exercise routine, worn-out shoes may be a factor. Place your old shoes on a table or other flat surface and look at them from the back. If they lean inward or outward or show signs of excessive wear, like badly worn edges of the sole, it's probably time for a new pair.

Reflect >>>> Reinforce >>>> Reinvigorate

Knowledge Check

Answers in Appendix D

1. The component(s) of physical fitness include:
   A. Cardiorespiratory endurance
   B. Muscular endurance
   C. Flexibility
   D. All of the above
2. The fourth level of the Physical Fitness Pyramid is reserved for:
   A. Muscular strength   B. Rest   C. Stretching
3. Less than ____ of adults achieve the recommended amount of regular physical activity.
   A. 16%   B. 39%   C. 50%

Modern Modifications

Try these suggestions when you find yourself becoming sedentary:

- Take breaks from long periods of sitting. Get up and stretch every 15 minutes. Walk across the room a few times.
- While watching television do a couple of simple exercises. Try sets of crunches, leg lifts, and/or modified push-ups during the commercials.
- While sitting in class or at a computer for an extended period of time, sit only on the front 6 inches of the seat, keeping your back straight. Correct posture will naturally engage your abs and other muscle groups as you sit.
- Do not use the remote. Get up to change the channels or turn the power on/off.

Critical Thinking

Answers in Appendix D

Scenario One: Mike has started going to the gym with his roommate. While lifting weights, Mike notices that his roommate can lift 30 lbs more than Mike can. Mike should not get discouraged because this disparity is due to:

A. Individual differences
B. Overload
C. Consistency

Scenario Two: Jim is on the track team. He used to stretch first thing when he went to practice, but recently his coach told the team that they should be stretching after their warm-ups. The coach changed the workout order because:

A. The team was too impatient to stretch before their warm-up
B. Stretching is safer when the muscles are warmer
C. Stretching is not an important aspect of a workout

Scenario Three: Amelia needs to buy a new pair of shoes for exercising. She has had a history of ankle sprains. She should find shoes that offer:

A. A wider toe box
B. Special arch support
C. A high-topped style that offers more ankle support

Going Above and Beyond

Websites

American Alliance for Health, Physical Education, Recreation, and Dance
http://www.aahperd.org

American College of Sports Medicine
http://www.acsm.org

American Council on Exercise
http://www.acefitness.org

American Heart Association
http://www.justmove.org

Canada's Physical Activity Guide
http://www.hc-sc.gc.ca/hppb/paguide

CDC Physical Activity Information
http://www.cdc.gov/nccdphp/phyactiv.htm

Health A to Z
http://www.healthatoz.com

Medicine and Science in Sports and Exercise
http://www.acsm-msse.org

MedlinePlus: Exercise and Physical Fitness
http://www.nlm.nih.gov/medlineplus/exercisephysicalfintess.html

Physician and Sports Medicine
http://www.physsportsmed.com

References and Suggested Readings

American College of Sports Medicine. *ACSM's Guidelines for Exercise Testing and Prescription*, Baltimore, MD: Lippincott Williams and Wilkins, 2000.

Balady G. J. Survival of the fittest—More evidence. *New England Journal of Medicine* 346(11)(2002): 852–854.

Blair S. N. et al. Is physical activity or physical fitness more important in defining health benefits? *Medicine and Science in Sports and Exercise* 33(6 Suppl)(2001): S379–S399.

Edlin, G. et al. *Health and Wellness, 7th Edition.* Sudbury, MA: Jones and Bartlett, 2002:142.

National Center for Chronic Disease Prevention and Health Promotion (NCCDPHP). *Components of Physical Fitness.* 2003. www.cdc.gov/nccdphp/dnpa/physical/components/index.htm [June 21, 2004].

NCCDPHP. *U.S. Physical Activity Statistics: 2001 State Summary Data.* 2001. http://apps.nccd.cdc.gov/PASurveillance/StateSumResultV.asp [June 18, 2004].

NCCDPHP. *Why Should I Be Active?* 2004. www.cdc.gov/nccdphp/dnpa/physical/importance/why.htm [June 18, 2004].

National Center for Health Statistics (NCHS) Vital Statistics System. *10 Leading Causes of Deaths, United States.* 2001. www.cdc.gov/ncipc/ [June 18, 2004].

Pescatello L. S. Exercising for health: the merits of lifestyle physical activity. *Western Journal of Medicine* 174(2)(2001):114–118.

Pfeiffer R. and Mangus B. *Concepts of Athletic Training, 4th Edition.* Sudbury, MA: Jones and Bartlett, 2004:265.

U.S. DHHS. *Healthy People 2010.* "The Healthy People 2010 Database, April 2004 Edition. http://wonder.cdc.gov/scripts/broker.exe [June 18, 2004].

U.S. DHHS. *Physical Activity and Health: A Report of the Surgeon General.* Atlanta, GA: DHHS, 1996.

CHAPTER 3

Improving Cardiorespiratory Endurance

Objectives

After reading this chapter, you should be able to:

- Differentiate between *aerobic* and *anaerobic* activities.
- Describe the benefits of cardiorespiratory exercises.
- Measure and assess your cardiorespiratory endurance.
- Design an appropriate cardiorespiratory exercise program.

Find the Beat: Determining Your Resting and Maximum Heart Rates

Your training heart rate zone is a critical element in exercise. Taking your pulse and checking your heart rate during a workout is one of the primary indicators to ascertain the intensity level at which you and your heart are working.

What Do I Need to Begin?

- An easy-to-read watch showing seconds
- A comfortable place to sit

How Do I Find My Pulse?

- **From your wrist at the radial artery.** Hold one hand in front of you, with your palm turned upward. Place your index and middle fingers on your wrist where your thumb and wrist meet. Feel for a strong beat.
- **On your neck at the carotid artery.** Place your index and middle fingers together and touch the Adam's apple. Slide your two fingers off of the Adam's apple into the groove beside it. Press gently and you should feel a beat. Pressing too hard or massaging this area on your neck can affect the heart rhythm.
- **Use an inexpensive watch-sized heart rate monitor.** The monitor does the work for you.
- Count your pulse for 10 seconds, then multiply that number by six. This will tell you the number of times your heart beats in a minute.

How Do I Find My Resting Heart Rate?

- To do this you must measure your heart rate when you first wake up in the morning before you get out of bed. Do this for 5 days.
- From these figures average the results.
- Measure your resting heart rate when you have had proper rest, a lack of stress, and proper nutrition. Remember that medication can also change your heart rate. If you are taking any kind of a sedative, antidepressant, or cold and flu medicine, this will likely alter your heart rate.

Resting Heart Rate Formula (Record in beats per minute):

Day 1 ( ) + Day 2 ( ) + Day 3 ( ) + Day 4 ( ) + Day 5 ( ) = ( ) ÷ 5 = ( ) Your Resting Heart Rate

How Do I Find My Maximum Heart Rate?

The easiest way to find your maximum heart rate is to subtract your age from 220.

Maximum Heart Rate Formula:

220 − ( ) (Your age) = ( ) Your Maximum Heart Rate

3

What's the word. . .

cardiorespiratory endurance activity
Exercise that contracts large muscle groups and increases breathing and heart rate.

aerobic exercise
Exercise that depends on oxygen for energy production.

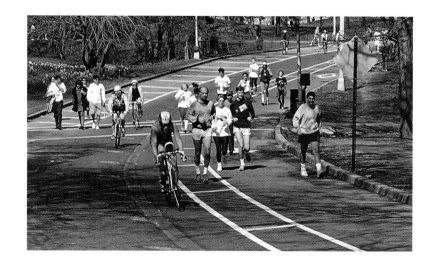

The Doorway to Cardiorespiratory Activity

From a health standpoint, **cardiorespiratory endurance activity** is about as close as you can get to an elixir for physical health and well-being. It can help you lose weight, ease stress, boost your immune system, and reduce the risk of certain diseases.

There are a few *buzz words* that are basically synonymous with cardiorespiratory activity:

- Cardiovascular activity
- Cardiopulmonary activity
- **Aerobic exercise**

Merriam-Webster's dictionary defines aerobic as "occurring only in the presence of oxygen." When linked with exercise, aerobic refers to any activity that increases oxygen intake and heart rate.

When you exercise aerobically:

- You repeatedly contract large muscle groups, such as your legs and arms.
- You increase your breathing and your heart rate.

Examples of aerobic exercises include:

- Walking (brisk pace)
- Jogging/running
- Bicycling: road or mountain
- In-line skating or rollerblading
- Swimming
- Cross-country skiing
- Treadmill
- Stationary bicycle
- Stair climber
- Rowing machine
- Aerobic dancing

Basic Physiology

The cardiorespiratory system is comprised of the following components:

- **Heart:** A muscle required to continuously deliver oxygen-rich blood to all the organs of the body.

- **Lungs:** Organs that provide the body with oxygen and rid the body of carbon dioxide through respiration.
- **Blood vessels:** A system of arteries, veins, and capillaries that transport blood to and from the heart.

Cardiovascular Processes

The processes of respiration and circulation (pulmonary and systemic) are all connected within the cardiovascular system. Working together, the heart, lungs, and blood vessels deliver and transport oxygen to the body without stopping. **Figure 3.1** outlines this intricate process in eight basic stages.

> **What's the word...**
>
> **pulmonary circulation**
> Circulation between the heart and the lungs.
>
> **systemic circulation**
> Circulation between the heart and the rest of the body.

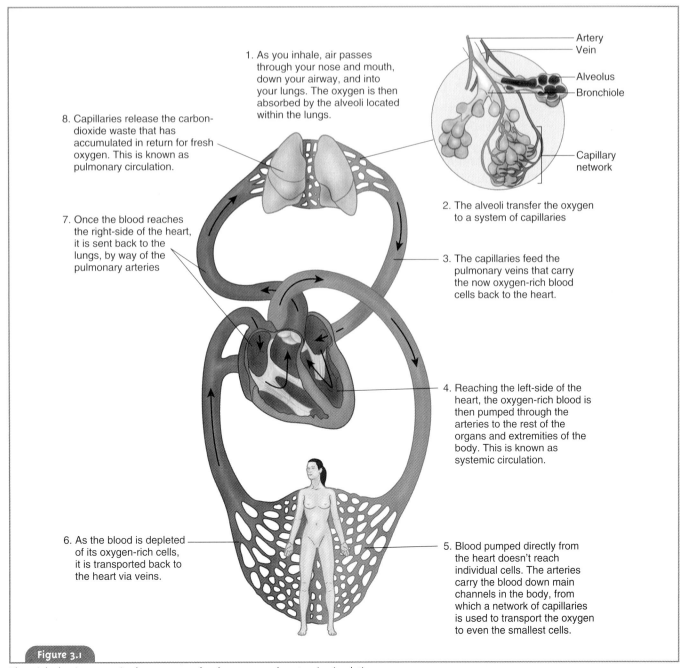

1. As you inhale, air passes through your nose and mouth, down your airway, and into your lungs. The oxygen is then absorbed by the alveoli located within the lungs.

8. Capillaries release the carbon-dioxide waste that has accumulated in return for fresh oxygen. This is known as pulmonary circulation.

Artery
Vein
Alveolus
Bronchiole
Capillary network

2. The alveoli transfer the oxygen to a system of capillaries

7. Once the blood reaches the right-side of the heart, it is sent back to the lungs, by way of the pulmonary arteries

3. The capillaries feed the pulmonary veins that carry the now oxygen-rich blood cells back to the heart.

4. Reaching the left-side of the heart, the oxygen-rich blood is then pumped through the arteries to the rest of the organs and extremities of the body. This is known as systemic circulation.

6. As the blood is depleted of its oxygen-rich cells, it is transported back to the heart via veins.

5. Blood pumped directly from the heart doesn't reach individual cells. The arteries carry the blood down main channels in the body, from which a network of capillaries is used to transport the oxygen to even the smallest cells.

Figure 3.1

The eight basic stages in the process of pulmonary and systemic circulation.

The ability of the body to deliver oxygen to and from the heart is critical. The more active you are, the more efficient your pulmonary and circulatory systems become. The less active one is, the weaker his or her heart muscle will be. Being sedentary and out of shape may have a more detrimental effect on one's health than other well-known risk factors such as smoking, high blood pressure, and heart disease (Myers 2002).

The basis of cardiorespiratory or aerobic training is to place greater demands on the heart than what is required during rest. By regularly overloading the heart in this fashion, it will become stronger. This results in the heart pumping more blood and delivering more oxygen to the body per heart beat, creating a lower resting heart rate. See the QuickStart on page 31 to determine your current resting heart rate.

Benefits of Cardiorespiratory Endurance Exercise

Regular endurance exercise can benefit the body in many healthy ways. Following are the short- and long-term benefits achieved by exercising regularly, using the cardiorespiratory system.

Short-Term Benefits

Many people start a physical activity program because of long-term benefits; however, it is the short-term benefits that keep them motivated to continue the habit.

Relaxes and Revitalizes

Physical activity reduces mental and muscular tension and increases concentration and energy levels. Regular aerobic exercise releases **endorphins**.

Increases Stamina

Exercise may cause fatigue immediately after the activity. Over the long term, though, it will increase stamina and reduce fatigue.

A Break from Daily Routine and Stress

Planned or unplanned physical activity can be enjoyable and a release from day-to-day stress and boredom.

Helps You Feel Good About Yourself

Physical activity can improve your self-esteem, self-confidence, and give you a general sense of well being.

Long-Term Benefits

Decreases Risk of Heart Disease

The American Heart Association (AHA) has identified physical *inactivity* as a risk factor for cardiovascular diseases—primarily heart attacks and strokes, which are the leading causes of death in the United States (American Heart Association [AHA] 1995).

Decreases Risk of Cancer

Physical activity lowers the risk of colon and breast cancer. Other types of cancers may also be lower in active people.

Lowers Blood Pressure

High blood pressure increases the risk of heart disease, stroke, and kidney disease. Inactive people are more likely to develop high blood pressure than those who are active. In addition, aerobic exercise can reduce the risks of high blood pressure.

The Inside Track

Before menopause, women have less cardiovascular disease than men do. After menopause, women's risk is closer to men's.

What's the word...

endorphins Protein produced in your brain that serves as your body's natural painkiller. Endorphins also reduce stress, depression, and anxiety.

obesity Excessive amounts of body fat.

type 2 diabetes A disease that involves the inability to produce an adequate amount of insulin.

The Inside Track

Women's bone density is typically greatest in their mid-20s to mid-30s, but then declines slowly until menopause, which becomes a time of rapid bone loss. Physical activity performed during younger years will help women maintain good bone mass at menopause. Even physical activity begun later in life or during menopause will help slow the loss of bone.

Lower Body Fat

Obesity is a risk factor for heart disease and a culprit in other diseases as well. Aerobic exercise preferentially burns fat, resulting in a decrease in total body fat.

Improves Muscular Health

Aerobic exercise stimulates the growth of blood vessels and capillaries in the muscles, providing for more efficient oxygen delivery to the muscles and helping to remove irritating metabolic waste products such as lactic acid. This can reduce pain in those who have fibromyalgia and chronic low-back pain.

Reduces Number of Sick Days

Many studies report that people who exercise regularly are less susceptible to minor viral illnesses, such as colds or flu, because of an improved immune system.

Decreases Chance of Premature Death

In 1986, results from the Harvard Alumni Health Study published in *New England Journal of Medicine* for the first time linked exercise with increased life spans. Since then, additional research has supported this finding.

Decreases Cholesterol and Triglyceride Levels

High blood cholesterol and triglyceride levels increase the risk of heart disease. Regular exercise raises the level of *good* cholesterol, or high-density lipoprotein (HDL), which may help clear blood vessels and lower the level of *bad* cholesterol, or low-density lipoprotein (LDL). HDLs and LDLs are discussed further in Chapter 6.

Decreases Risk of Diabetes

Physical activity lowers the risk of type 2 diabetes, and because it helps regulate blood sugar, it can decrease the need for drugs in those who already have **type 2 diabetes** (AHA 2004b).

Decreases Risk of Osteoporosis

Gradual bone loss that may lead to fractures can be delayed by regular exercise. Exercise also is known to promote bone formation.

Decreases Arthritis Symptoms

Regular exercise helps keep joints flexible and helps build muscle to support the joint.

Assessing Cardiorespiratory Fitness/Endurance

Cardiorespiratory fitness or endurance is largely determined by habitual physical activity. As defined earlier in the chapter, aerobic, or cardiorespiratory, exercise involves oxygen. When you assess your cardiorespiratory endurance, you are actually measuring how efficiently your system is using oxygen.

Maximal Oxygen Uptake

Determining maximal oxygen uptake (VO_{2max}):
- Is the best measure of cardiorespiratory fitness
- Reveals how efficiently the cardiorespiratory system uses oxygen
- Requires an exercise physiology laboratory with trained personnel to analyze a person's oxygen intake

Maximal tests can be substituted with submaximal tests, which are a comparable way to score the VO_{2max} as they are less expensive, require little to no equipment, and are, therefore, more practical.

Submaximal Tests

Submaximal tests can give a fairly good estimate of VO_{2max}.
- Monitoring your heart rate is necessary for these tests.
- Large numbers of people can be tested at one time.
- These tests require little equipment.
- Test results can be affected by a person's motivation and pacing ability.

The following tests are commonly used to judge cardiorespiratory endurance. The instructions for each are provided in the corresponding lab.
- *1-Mile Walking Test (Lab 3.2, Activity 1)*
- *YMCA Step Test (Lab 3.2, Activity 3)*
- *1.5-mile Run/Walk Test (Lab 3.2, Activity 2)*

Please complete Lab 2.1 before taking any of these tests.

Designing a Cardiorespiratory Endurance Exercise Program

Every person has individual needs. Your exercise program should consist of physical activities that are right for your body, your endurance level, and specifically make you feel good, both mentally and physically. As you proceed with your program make sure you:
- Warm up and cool down
- Follow the FITT guidelines
- Progress safely

Warm-Up

Begin each exercise session with a warm-up.
- Usually the warm-up is done by doing the same activity as the workout, but at a low intensity.
- You can also simply swing your arms from side to side for a couple minutes or walk around at a steady pace.

What's the word...

maximal oxygen uptake (VO_{2max}) How efficiently the cardiorespiratory system uses oxygen.

The Inside Track

A common mistake is stretching before muscles are warmed up. Not only is it difficult to stretch cold muscles, but there are risks to exercising heavily on muscles that are not warm, especially as you get older.

- After 5 to 10 minutes, stretch the primary muscles used in the warm-up before proceeding to the cardiorespiratory endurance exercise.

Cool-Down

End each exercise session with a cool-down.
- The cool-down should last 5–10 minutes and be done at a low intensity.
- Allow your heart rate, breathing, and circulation to return to normal.
- Again, stretch the primary muscles used.

FITT Guidelines

After the warm-up, the FITT guidelines are an easy way to remember the essential facts for a good and effective aerobic exercise (Table 3.1).

Frequency

The American College of Sports Medicine (2000) recommends exercising three to five days each week within the target heart rate zone for cardiorespiratory fitness. More frequent exercising provides few additional benefits and may increase the likelihood of injury. Significant fitness loss occurs within two weeks of becoming inactive.

Intensity

There are several ways to monitor exercise intensity. Five popular methods include:
- Maximum heart rate method
- Heart rate reserve method using the Karvonen Formula
- Rate of perceived exertion method
- Calories burned
- Talk-test method

The Inside Track

Those who are considered obese should avoid vigorous-intensity workouts and should consult a doctor before beginning an exercise regimen.

Table 3.1	Aerobic FITT Guidelines	
Frequency	Start with 3 days per week and work up to 5 days per week. More than 5 days per week can lead to injury and is not necessary for promoting health.	
Intensity	Based on maximum heart rate: 70 to 85%	Based on heart rate reserve: 60 to 80%
Time	20 to 60 minutes, within your target heart rate zone	

Type	Choose an aerobic activity that:
	    Increases breathing, elevates heart rate, and maintains that heart rate level for an extended period
	    Uses repetitive, rhythmic, large-muscle movements performed continuously over an extended time
	Start-and-stop sports such as tennis, racquetball, and basketball are also aerobic, if skill levels allow continuous play and are intense enough to raise heart rate to target levels.	

Source: Adapted from American College of Sports Medicine.

The Inside Track
Resting between high-intensity workouts is essential to prevent injury and to promote recovery.

What's the word. . .

target heart rate zone A range of heart rates used to maintain optimal effects during aerobic exercise.

pulse The surge of blood that can be felt on certain points on the body each time the heart pumps blood into the arteries.

rate of perceived exertion A person's own perception of the intensity of his or her exercise.

Both the maximum heart rate and heart rate reserve methods are heart rate-based measurements. They work by measuring increases in heart rate. These methods provide a quick and easy way to gauge the intensity of your workout. However, an increase in heart rate is not the training stimulus; heart rate increase is only indicative of oxygen consumption required during the exercise.

Maximum Heart Rate Method

According to the American College of Sports Medicine (ACSM), you should exercise using 70% to 85% of your maximum heart rate. To calculate your maximum heart rate, refer to the Quick Start on page 31. To find your target heart rate zone, multiply your maximum heart rate (MHR) by 70% (low end of the range) and 85% (high end of the range).

Maximum HR _____ × 70% = _____ *Low End of Target Zone*
Maximum HR _____ × 85% = _____ *High End of Target Zone*

Take your pulse during your workout to determine if the intensity of the exercise has increased your heart rate to the target zone.

Calculating Heart Rate Reserve (HRR) Using the Karvonen Formula

For this method you will need to calculate both your resting and maximum heart rates. Begin by finding your maximum heart rate, then subtract your resting heart rate from that number.

Maximum HR _____ − *Resting HR* _____ = _____ *New Value*

The American College of Sports Medicine recommends a target range of 60% to 80%. So, multiply the new value by 60% (low end of the range) and 80% (high end of the range).

New Value _____ × 60% = _____ *Low End of Target Zone*
New Value _____ × 80% = _____ *High End of Target Zone*

Rate of Perceived Exertion

A person's own perception of the intensity of his or her exercise can often be as accurate as the heart rate in gauging exercise intensity. Measurements are based on a 20-point scale. Six is no exertion and twenty is maximum exertion. The Borg scale shown in Figure 3.2 lets you determine your rate of perceived exertion (RPE). This scale consists of numerical ratings for physical exercise followed by their associated descriptive ratings (Borg 1982). To judge perceived exertion:

- Estimate how difficult it feels to do the exercise.
- Do not be concerned with any one single factor such as shortness of breath or work intensity.
- Concentrate on the total inner feeling of exertion.
- Multiplying the rating of perceived exertion by 10 roughly approximates the heart rate during exercise. These numbers were chosen because when multiplied by ten, they roughly equal the resting and maximum heart rate values of 60 and 200 beats per minute, respectively.

  For example, Mary Susan perceives she is exerting a 14 while dancing in her Scottish dance class. She multiplies that by 10. This estimates Mary Susan's heart rate for this kind of exercise should be at or around 140.

- Once accustomed to a particular exercise, you will be able to estimate your heart rate based on your RPE. Most people should workout at a perceived exertion between 12 and 15.

Calories—Not Just Used for Dieting

Calories per hour is the amount of energy an exerciser expends when maintaining the same exercise intensity for an hour. This value is calculated by most exercise machines and pedometers.

The Borg RPE Scale

6	No exertion at all
7	Extremely light
8	
9	Very light
10	
11	Light
12	
13	Somewhat hard
14	
15	Hard (heavy)
16	
17	Very hard
18	Extremely hard
19	
20	Maximal exertion

Figure 3.2

The Borg RPE Scale. Rating of perceived exertion (RPE) can be used to monitor your response to physical activity. (*Source:* For correct usage of the scale, the user must go to the instruction and administration given by Borg, see Borg, G. 1998. *Borg's Perceived Exertion and Pain Scales.* Champaign, IL: Human Kinetics, or to the folder published by Borg on the RPE scale or the CR10 scale, Borg Perception, Furuholmen 1027, 762 91 Rimbo, Sweden.)

Talk-Test Method

The talk-test method of measuring intensity is simple. A person who is active at a light-intensity level should be able to talk while doing the activity. One who is active at a moderate-intensity level should be able to carry on a conversation comfortably while engaging in the activity. If a person becomes winded or too out of breath to carry on a conversation, the activity can be considered vigorous.

Determining the Appropriate Intensity for Your Workout

Now that you have calculated your target zone. Determining the intensity level at which you should exercise is quite simple. The ACSM says that exercising at 70% to 85% MHR or 60% to 80% HRR for 20 to 30 minutes, excluding the time spent warming up and cooling down, enables most individuals to achieve good health, fitness, and weight management goals. Your individual level of fitness will ultimately determine where you fall within this range.

When starting an exercise program, aim at the lowest value of your target zone during the first few weeks. Gradually build up to the higher values of your target zone—this may take at least 1 month or up to 6 months or more. The ACSM recommends that healthy adults gradually advance or progress in a cardiorespiratory exercise program to avoid muscle aches, pain, and discouragement.

You should always be able to catch your breath and speak comfortably while exercising. Feeling effort or maybe even slight discomfort is normal during some exercise. You should, however, never sense pain. Always warm up slowly and cool down gradually.

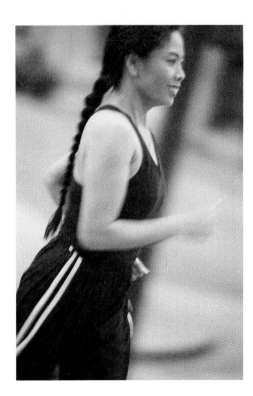

Table 3.2	Comparing Intensity of Physical Activity		
Intensity	Heart Rate Reserve (HRR) %	Maximal Heart Rate (MHR) %	Rating of Perceived Exertion (RPE)
Very light	<25	<30	<9
Light	25–44	30–49	9–10
Moderate	45–59	50–69	11–12
Hard	60–84	80–89	13–16
Very hard	>85	>90	>16
Maximal	100	100+	20

Source: Adapted from Public Health Service. *Surgeon General's Report on Physical Activity and Health.* Washington, D.C.: U.S. Government Printing Office, 1996.

The Correlation Between Frequency and Intensity

Exercise classified as moderate or Level 1 in the Physical Activity Pyramid is recommended on a daily basis. If your goal is to:

- Maintain or improve general fitness—exercise at an intensity of moderate to hard
- Maintain or increase performance-related fitness—occasionally exercise at an intensity of hard to very hard

Exercise intensities of extremely hard to maximal should only be performed by individuals in excellent aerobic condition. Exercise in this range cannot be sustained for long time periods and is primarily performed to develop the anaerobic energy system and improve performance in activities such as sprinting. **Table 3.2** describes the relationship of exercise intensity to HRR, MHR, and RPE.

Time or Duration of Exercise

A cardiorespiratory endurance session should vary from 20–60 minutes (single session or several sessions of 10 or more minutes each) to gain significant aerobic and fat-burning benefits. This does not include the warm-up and cool-down phases of your program. All beginners, especially those who are out of shape, should take a very conservative approach and train at relatively low intensities for 10–25 minutes. As you get into better shape, you can gradually increase the duration of time you exercise.

Gradually increase the duration of exercise, before you increase the intensity. For example, when beginning a brisk walking program, be more concerned with increasing the number of minutes of the exercise session before you increase how fast you walk or add a hilly terrain.

Type of Aerobic Activities

To choose the best exercises for you, consider the following:

- Choose exercise that involves several muscle groups and that is weight bearing. This will require the greatest amount of energy and oxygen to perform.
- Choose exercises that you enjoy the most.
- Alleviate boredom and decrease your risk for injuries by cross-training or alternating the types of exercise you perform.

Table 3.3 provides a few choices of indoor and outdoor aerobic activities, and the pros and cons of why you may or may not choose one of these activities for your exercise.

Table 3.3	Types of Indoor and Outdoor Aerobic Activity	
Activity	Pros	Cons
Walking 	• Most popular of all activities • No age limit—a lifetime activity • Convenient • Easily incorporated into lifestyle • Little skill involved • No cost • Fewer injuries than jogging or running • You can take in seasonal changes or walk through city streets and people watch • This is a weight-bearing exercise • Uses most major lower body muscle groups	• Not active enough for some • Takes three times longer to get the same aerobic benefit as from running • Injuries can occur, such as shin splints and blisters
Jogging/running 	• Convenient • High levels of cardiorespiratory fitness benefits in short time periods • Few skills needed • Impact on hard surface builds stronger bones and offers protection against osteoporosis • Euphoric feeling or "runner's high" • In bad weather, you can run on an indoor track, if one is available • Low cost—just need a good pair of running shoes • Because it is often done outdoors, you get to view nature and a change of scenery	• Frequent, chronic injuries from impact to muscles, tendons, ligaments, and bones • Injuries such as shin splints and stress fractures due to: • Improper warm-up • Excessive distances • Impact of feet and legs on ground • Wearing inadequate shoes • Dangerous when done on roads with traffic • Poor outdoor conditions (i.e., snow, pollution) may prohibit
Bicycling: road or mountain 	• No age limit—a lifetime activity • Fewer injuries than running because there is less impact on legs and feet • Because it is done outdoors, you get to view nature and a change of scenery	• May be difficult to locate a safe place to ride • Injuries include painful knees, feet, back, and saddle soreness • Cost for the bike and other gear such as helmet, gloves, water bottle, sunscreen, and glasses

continues

Table 3.3	Types of Indoor and Outdoor Aerobic Activity, *continued*	
Activity	**Pros**	**Cons**
In-line skating or rollerblading	• Lots of fun—curving, turning, gliding, sprinting, and spinning • Change of scenery • Works thighs, hips, and buttocks muscles	• There is a learning curve, which could make the beginning stages a bit dangerous • May be difficult to locate a safe place to skate • Some people have difficulty stopping • Injuries may result from collisions, falling, and blisters • Requires skill and balance • Coasting loses the aerobic effects • Costs for skates, helmet, wrist guards, knee guards, elbow guards, and gloves

Swimming	• Fewer injuries because there is no impact on legs and feet
	• Good for people who are
	  • injured and want to keep exercising
	  • pregnant
	  • overweight
	• Works every part of the body, with an emphasis on the upper body
	• Refreshing
	• No age limit—lifetime activity
		• You must locate a swimming pool and an available lane for swimming laps
		• Requires skill
		• Repetitive arm motions can result in pain and inflammation, leading to tendonitis and bursitis
		• Swimming laps can be repetitive and seem boring
		• Not a social activity
		• Since this exercise doesn't involve impact, it does not help build bone density
		• Risk of infections in the ears, eyes, and sinus

Cross-country skiing	• Involves both lower and upper body, including most major muscle groups when poles are used • Rigorous workout obtained when at higher altitudes, in cold weather, and added weight of clothing • Scenery changes • Low impact	• Exposure to cold conditions can lead to frostnip, frostbite, or hypothermia • Requires accessibility to snow • Skiing downhill decreases the aerobic effect

Table 3.3	Types of Indoor and Outdoor Aerobic Activity, *continued*	
Activity	Pros	Cons
Treadmill	• Easily accessible no matter what the weather conditions • Good for beginners, many levels • Easy to use • Easier on joints than walking or jogging on asphalt and concrete surfaces • Can watch TV while exercising • Some machines have various personal high-tech computer programs that monitor heart rate	• Can get monotonous • Can stumble and slide off • Expensive to own; may require health club membership
Stationary bicycle	• Great thigh workout • Gives knees a rest • Can read or watch TV while exercising • Easy to use	• With stationary bikes you have added convenience, but lose the ability to ride outdoors • Expensive to own; may require health club membership

continues

Table 3.3	Types of Indoor and Outdoor Aerobic Activity, *continued*	
Activity	Pros	Cons
Rowing machine	• Total body workout using most major muscle groups • Can watch TV while exercising • Will prepare you for outdoor rowing or paddling on a canoe or kayak	• Can strain back if not performed correctly • Repetitive motion can become boring • Requires coordination

Aerobic dancing	• Enjoyable
	 • Can be done with a class or individually at home with a video or a televised class
	 • Camaraderie can develop within a group of people working out together
	 • Low injury rates
	 • Different styles and variations of classes may be classified as below:
	   - High impact—more jumping and faster movement
	   - Low impact—less jumping and slower movement
	   - Aquatic—done in the water
	   - Step-aerobics using a 6"–12" step—increase impact and weight-bearing movement
	   - Kick boxing—uses movements of kick boxing for added variety and strength
	   - Circuit—uses weights and aerobics to work out upper body as well as to increase aerobic endurance
		• Possible injuries could occur, such as shin splints, tendonitis, muscle strain, back strain, and stress fracture
		 • Cost of class or travel time to a gym

Progression

There is a tendency when first beginning a fitness regimen for people to do too much too quickly. Keep in mind that just because you don't meet your goal the first day doesn't mean that you won't get there eventually. Slow and consistent improvement is the safe way to train.

If you have been sedentary, begin by doing a brisk walk or by bouncing on an exercise ball for 5 to 10 minutes. Gradually increase the duration of the activity by 10% per

Table 3.4	Progression for Cardiorespiratory Exercise			
Program stage	Week #	Frequency (days/week)	Intensity (% HRR)	Time (minutes)
Initial stage	1	3	40–50	15–20
	2	3–4	40–50	20–25
	3	3–4	50–60	20–25
	4	3–4	50–60	25–30
Improvement stage	5–7	3–4	60–70	25–30
	8–10	3–4	60–70	30–35
	11–13	3–4	65–75	30–35
	14–16	3–5	65–75	30–35
	17–20	3–5	70–85	35–40
	21–24	3–5	70–85	35–40
Maintenance stage	24+	3–5	70–85	30–45

Source: Adapted from American College of Sports Medicine. *ACSM's Guidelines for Exercise Testing and Prescription*, Philadelphia: Lippincott Williams and Wilkins, 2000.

week until you can perform 20 to 60 minutes continuously. Your training intensity during these exercise sessions should be between 70% and 85% of the maximum heart rate.

Reference **Table 3.4** for the American College of Sports Medicine's recommendations on how to progress in a cardiorespiratory exercise program.

Rules for Progression

1. Increase only one FITT component at a time. It is best to increase duration first.
2. Increase your exercise workout by no more than 10% per week. Increasing too fast will lead to injury.
3. Stop exercising and seek immediate health care if you experience any of the following:
- Tightness in your chest
- Severe shortness of breath
- Chest pain or pain in your arms or jaw, often on the left side
- Heart palpitations
- Dizziness, faintness, or feeling sick to your stomach

Conclusion

Aerobic activity can increase your overall wellness by boosting your immune system, easing stress, improving your self-image, and reducing the risk of certain diseases. When you exercise, you strengthen your heart, making it more efficient to pump oxygen-rich blood to the rest of the body. Submaximal tests assess how efficiently the cardiorespiratory system uses oxygen.

When designing your fitness program, make sure to follow the FITT guidelines. Always warm up and cool down, and progress slowly. Choose activities that are appropriate for your fitness level, patience, interests, and schedule. Most importantly, have fun!

Reflect >>>> Reinforce >>>> Reinvigorate

Knowledge Check

Answers in Appendix D

1. Circulation between the heart and lungs is called . . .
   A. Pulmonary circulation
   B. Systemic circulation
   C. Cardiovascular circulation
2. What does aerobic mean?
   A. Exercising with a pain in your chest
   B. Exercising using oxygen
   C. Exercising for more than 60 minutes
3. The body's natural painkiller that is produced in the brain is . . .
   A. Histamine
   B. Endorphins
   C. Oxygen

Modern Modifications

Try a couple of these suggestions to add a little more heart-friendly activity to your daily routine:

- Park at the farthest spot in the parking lot and walk briskly or jog to the door.
- Take the stairs—avoid the escalator and elevator as much as possible.
- Turn up the stereo and dance. Cut loose for a couple of minutes when your favorite song comes on the radio.
- When shopping, walk the length of the mall between entering stores.
- Put away the leaf-blower and snow-blower—pick up a rake or shovel instead.
- After you take the dog for a walk, stay outside and play with the dog for an extra 30 minutes.
- Join an intramural team. It's great exercise, you meet new people, and it is a fun way to spend a couple of hours!

Critical Thinking

Answers in Appendix D

Scenario One: Gary is 18 years old and would like to improve his cardiorespiratory health. What should be his first step toward putting together an effective exercise program?

A. Take a submaximal test to find his current cardiorespiratory fitness level
B. Begin running 2 miles a week
C. Bike for 40 minutes a day and gradually add in other activities

Scenario Two: Marcia is 23 years old and has been told that stretching is an important component to cardiorespiratory training. When is the best time for Marcia to stretch?

A. First thing when she gets to the gym

B. 50 minutes after exercising, when her muscles have cooled down

C. After she warms up for 5–10 minutes and before she starts her routine

Scenario Three: Sylvia is 20 years old, walks 15 minutes a day, and would like to increase her level of activity. What is the safest way for Sylvia to progress with her cardiorespiratory training?

A. Jog for the 15 minutes instead of walking

B. Increase the duration of her walks by 10% each week until she feels comfortable walking for 60 minutes continuously

C. Try running a mile once a week in addition to her daily walks

Going Above and Beyond

Websites

American Academy of Orthopedic Surgeons
http://orthinfo.asos.org

American Heart Association
http://www.americanheart.org or *http://www.justmove.org*

Cooper Institute for Aerobics Research
http://www.cooperinst.org

MedlinePlus: Exercise and Physical Fitness
http://www.nlm.nih.gov/medlineplus/exercisephysicalfitness.html

Physician and Sports Medicine
http://www.physsportmed.com

Runner's World Online
http://www.runnersworld.com

Shape up America! Fitness Center
http://shapeup.org/fitness

Walking
http://walking.miningco.com

References and Suggested Readings

American College of Sports Medicine. ACSM position stand: the recommended quantity and quality of exercise for developing and maintaining cardiorespiratory, muscular fitness and flexibility in healthy adults. *Medicine and Science in Sports and Exercise 30*(6)(1998): 975–991.

American College of Sports Medicine. *ACSM's Guidelines for Exercise Testing and Prescription*, Philadelphia: Lippincott Williams and Wilkins, 2000.

American Heart Association. A statement on exercise: benefits and recommendations for physical activity programs for all americans. *Circulation 91*(1995): 580.

American Heart Association (AHA). "Cholesterol." 2004a. *http://www.americanheart.org* [June 14, 2004].

AHA. "Diabetes Mellitus." 2004b. *http://www.americanheart.org* [June 14, 2004].

AHA. "Resting Heart Rate." 2004c. *http://www.americanheart.org* [June 14, 2004].

AHA. "Target Heart Rate." 2004d. *http://www.americanheart.org* [June 14, 2004].

Blair S. N. and Jackson A. S. Physical fitness and activity as separate heart disease risk factors: a meta-analysis. *Medicine and Science in Sports and Exercise 33*(5)(2001): 762–764.

Borg G. A. Psychophysical basis of perceived exertion, *Medicine and Science in Sports and Exercise 14*(1982): 377.

Carroll J. F. and Kyser C. K. Exercise training in obesity lowers blood pressure independent of weight change. *Medicine and Science in Sports and Exercise 34*(4)(2002): 596–601.

Cooper K. H. *The Aerobics Program for Well-Being.* Toronto: Bantam Books, 1982.

Erikssen G, Physical fitness and changes in mortality: the survival of the fittest. *Sports Medicine 31*(8)(2001): 571–576.

Fletcher G. et al. American Heart Association: statement on exercise. *Circulation 86*(1992): 2726.

Merriam-Webster Dictionary. "aerobic" and "obesity." 2004. *http://www.merriam-webster.com* [June 14, 2004].

Myers J. et al. Exercise capacity and mortality among men referred for exercise testing. *New England Journal of Medicine 346*(1)(2002): 793–801.

Public Health Service. *Surgeon General's Report on Physical Activity and Health.* Washington, D.C.: U.S. Government Printing Office, 1996.

UC Davis Health System. "The Well-Connected Report- Exercise" March 2000. *http://wellness.ucdavis.edu/wellconnected/exercise29.html* [June 14, 2004].

CHAPTER 4

Increasing Flexibility

Objectives

After reading this chapter, you should be able to:

- Define flexibility and describe the benefits of increased flexibility.
- Explain the factors influencing flexibility.
- Assess flexibility.
- Explain the difference between ballistic, static, dynamic, and proprioceptive neuromuscular facilitation (PNF) stretching.
- Describe various types of stretching exercises.
- Implement stretching into an exercise program.
- Explain how low-back pain can be prevented.
- Describe which exercises can help prevent back pain.
- List the ways to improve your posture.

How Can You Motivate Yourself to Stretch?

Incorporate a stretching workout program into your daily schedule.

Make Stretching Fun

Listen to music, visit with a friend, meditate, or watch television while stretching.

Stretches You Can Do Anytime

Tear out and tape in front of your desk the following list of exercises:

1. Clasp your hands together and stretch out in front of you.

2. In the same position, stretch your hands over your head.

3. Lean right.

4. Lean left.

5. Clasp your hands behind your back and open up your chest area.

6. Stretch your wrists by bending your wrists back, then down, then in a circle.

7. Lift your shoulders up to your ears, then down and back. Do that five times.

8. Take your right hand and put it on your left shoulder. With your left hand, gently push your right elbow, pushing your right hand past your shoulder and stretching the back of your right arm.

9. Stretch your left arm in the same manner.

10. Put your hands flat on your desk, palms down, and push your chair out, stretching your back.

11. Feel free to add more stretches for a variety and to avoid boredom! Remember, SIT UP STRAIGHT! Good posture starts now!

Keep Track of Your Progress

From time to time, use the tests in the lab and in the chapter to assess your flexibility.

What Are the Benefits of Flexibility?

Flexibility offers the following benefits:
- Increases joint movement (mobility)
- Improves circulation, bringing nutrients to keep tissues healthy and transporting wastes out of the tissues
- Improves performance in some activities
- Improves posture and personal appearance
- Valuable during the cool-down phase of a workout
- Prevents low-back problems
- Improves coordination and balance, which helps maintain an independent and active lifestyle in the elderly
- Helps reduce excess stress by lowering anxiety and boosting feelings of self-confidence

What's the word. . .

flexibility Ability to move a joint smoothly through a full range of motion.

stretching Primary method of improving flexibility.

static or passive stretching Muscle is stretched naturally without force being applied.

dynamic or active stretching Muscle is taken beyond its normal range of motion with help from a partner.

What Determines Flexibility?

- Flexibility is an important part of physical fitness, but it is often overlooked during workouts.
- Flexibility is achieved by **stretching**. Stress causes muscles to contract and tighten. Stretching helps muscles relax, relieving pain from muscular stress.
- There are two kinds of stretching: **static** and **dynamic**.

Factors That Influence Flexibility

- *Muscle temperature.* Warm muscles stretch more easily than cold muscles.
- *Physical activity.* Sedentary individuals are less flexible; active individuals tend to maintain or even increase flexibility.
- *Injury.* Injury can limit range of motion, but a good rehabilitation program can help regain all or part of a joint's flexibility.
- *Body composition.* Most muscular individuals have good flexibility because they have trained their muscles through a full range of motion. Overly bulky muscles may limit movement (known as being "muscle bound"), but this is rare. Fat can also limit movement and flexibility.
- *Age.* As a person ages, flexibility declines due more to inactivity than the aging process itself. Flexibility can be maintained by doing stretching activities regularly.
- *Disease.* Diseases such as arthritis can make it uncomfortable or even painful to move joints. Arthritic individuals can improve joint mobility through exercise.

Assessing Flexibility

You cannot determine flexibility with one test since the flexibility of one joint does not indicate flexibility in other joints.

Precautions

Take the following precautions when testing your flexibility:

1. Warm up before doing a test.
2. Stop the test if pain occurs.
3. Do not perform fast, jerky movements.
4. If any of the following apply, seek medical advice before performing a test:
   a. Presently suffering from acute back pain
   b. Currently receiving treatment for back pain
   c. Ever had a surgical operation on your back
   d. Health-care professional told you never to exercise your back

Sit-and-Reach Test

Step 1: Sit on the floor with your legs straight, knees together, and toes pointing toward the ceiling.

Step 2: Place one hand over the other. Place tips of two middle fingers on top of each other.

Step 3: Slowly stretch forward without bouncing or jerking. Stop when you feel tightness or discomfort in your back or legs.

Step 4: Repeat the test three more times. Record your score by using ⬤ Table 4.1 .
Record your scores as follows:

First attempt: _____ points

Second attempt: _____ points

Third attempt: _____ points

Total points =   _____ divided by 3 = _____ **your score**

Score your results by averaging your three attempts.

Table 4.1	Scoring Results for the Sit-and-Reach Test
If you reached . . .	**You get . . .**
more than two inches past your toes	1 point - excellent
to your toes and up to two inches past	2 points - good
up to four inches from your toes	3 points - fair
more than four inches from your toes	4 points - poor

Source: Imrie D. and Barbuto L. *Back Power.* Toronto: Stoddart, 1988.

4

Table 4.2	Scoring Results for the Shoulder Flexibility Test
If . . .	**Your flexibility is . . .**
you can clasp your hands together	very good.
your fingertips almost touch	good, but needs work.
you are not within an inch of touching your fingertips together	poor; needs a lot of work.

Source: Imrie D. and Barbuto L. *Back Power.* Toronto: Stoddart, 1988.

Shoulder Flexibility Test

Step 1: Bring your right hand over your shoulder and down between your shoulder blades.

Step 2: Bring your left hand around the small of your back and up between your shoulder blades.

Step 3: Try to touch the fingertips of both hands behind your back.

Step 4: Have someone measure the distance between your fingertips.

Step 5: Do the test the other way: left hand over your head and down between your shoulder blades, right hand reaching behind your back up to your shoulder blades.

Step 6: Try to touch the fingertips of both hands behind your back.

Step 7: Have someone measure the distance between your fingertips.

Score your results using (Table 4.2).

Other Flexibility Tests

There are many other tests that can be used to assess your flexibility. See Lab 4.1, Activity 3 for additional flexibility assessments.

What's the word. . .

stretch reflex An involuntary muscle contraction against a quick stretch.

The Inside Track

Physiology of Stretching

Areas within your muscles and tendons protect them from overstretching or tearing during a quick stretch by creating a **stretch reflex**. For example, someone tapping your leg just below the kneecap quickly stretches the quadriceps muscle. This makes your thigh contract and kick out your lower leg. The quicker the stretch, the stronger the reflex.

The protective action of tendons causes a stretched muscle attached to the tendon to relax, and signal its opposing muscle to contract. This protects the stretched muscle and tendon from tearing.

By stretching slowly during exercise, you avoid contracting the muscle you are trying to stretch. As a stretch is held, your muscles and tendons adapt to the new length.

Maintain Your Flexibility: Do Regular Stretching Workouts

- The adage "use it or lose it" applies especially to flexibility.
- Do a brief (5 to 10 minute) warm-up such as jogging in place, brisk walking, or riding a stationary bicycle. Do not stretch to warm up, but warm up to stretch. Stretching while muscles are cold may injure muscles. Warming up gradually increases your heart rate and blood flow and raises the temperature of muscles, ligaments, and tendons.
- Stretch all the major muscle groups in the body (arms, shoulders, chest, back, legs).
- Do not stretch swollen joints.
- Stretch the muscle group slowly, until slight discomfort is felt (not pain).
- Do not hold your breath—breathe normally.

- Do not bounce at the end of a stretch.
- Hold the stretch for at least 10 to 30 seconds.
- Repeat the stretch four times.
- A workout to stretch all of the major joints will last 10 to 15 minutes.
- Do all at once or piecemeal throughout the day.
- Stretch at least 2 to 3 days per week; every day is okay.
- Cool down after stretching. Warm muscles stretch better and their range of motion increases. The greatest improvements in flexibility come after exercising.

Types of Stretching

Stretching techniques include static stretches, ballistic stretches, and PNF (proprioceptive neuromuscular facilitation).

Static Stretching

Static stretching is the most practical type of stretching. It is effective, causes less pain, and is usually easier to do.

Perform a static stretch by:

1. Slowly and gently stretch the muscle to the point of discomfort and hold that position for 10–30 seconds.
2. Slightly back off and, while holding this position, relax.
3. Take a deep breath and exhale.
4. Slowly and gently stretch again to the point of discomfort (this point should be beyond the first step).

See Table 4.3 for proper stretching exercises and Table 4.4 for potentially harmful exercises that should be avoided.

Ballistic Stretching

Ballistic stretching uses bouncing, repetitive movements to force a stretch past the normal range of motion.

Tipping Point

Rewards
- Avoid **ballistic stretching**; for example, bending forcefully to touch your toes with your knees straight and bouncing while you reach. Ballistic stretching may do more harm than good, because the muscles may shorten reflexively. This type of stretching is not recommended for most people. However, some athletes believe that controlled ballistic stretching can better prepare a muscle for sustained activity, especially one requiring a burst of speed.

What's the word. . .

ballistic stretching
Bouncing, repetitive movement during stretching.

Table 4.3 | Proper Form for Stretching Exercises

Neck

Ear to shoulder   Chin to chest   Look right and left

Shoulders, chest, upper back, and abdominals

Shoulder roll   Back scratch   Handcuff stretch   Rack

Reach up   Slow arm circles   Arm across chest   Wall press

Hamstrings, groin, lower back

Supine hamstring stretch

Modified hurdler

Single knee to chest

Double knee to chest

Calf

Quads, inner thigh, hips

Standing heel-to-buttock
(do not perform without your
health-care provider's advice if you
have knee pain or knee surgery)

Standing lunge

Side (skater) lunge

Butterfly

Table 4.4	Potentially Harmful Exercises to Avoid

Full squat: Strain on the knees

Plough: Strain on the neck, shoulders, and spine

Double leg raises: Strain on the spine; can cause injury to disks

Full neck circles: Strain on neck

Standing toe touch: Strain on lower back and knees

Hurdler's stretch

Hands behind head sit-up

Stresses the knee joint by placing the knee in an unnatural position.

Creates stress on the cervical spine. Best to place hands over the ears or fold arms across chest. Perform curl-ups or crunches.

Proprioceptive Neuromuscular Facilitation

Proprioceptive neuromuscular facilitation (PNF) involves tightening a muscle as hard as you can right before you stretch it. The theory behind PNF is that the act of tightening or squeezing exhausts the muscle so that it becomes relaxed and more receptive to the stretch.

PNF may be the most effective type of stretching (static stretching is almost as good), but it usually requires a partner, takes more time, and can cause more muscle soreness. There are several PNF techniques. An example of one method of performing a PNF stretch follows:

- Do a near-maximum 6-second isometric contraction of the muscle you wish to stretch.
- Immediately relax the muscle for 2 seconds, then have a partner push the muscle into a static stretch for 10 to 15 seconds.

Back Fitness

Over 80% of North Americans suffer back pain in their lifetime. Low-back pain, both acute and chronic, centers on the muscles supporting the spine. Age and physical condition are the major factors associated with low-back pain, along with the trauma of lifting something in the wrong way, or injuring yourself in an activity or sport. Being overweight, poor posture, stress, and occupation (e.g., computer programmers and truck drivers) contribute to the pain. There is also recent research indicating a link between smoking and lower back pain.

Preventing Low-back Pain

To prevent low-back pain:

- Exercise regularly to improve the strength of your back and abdominal muscles.
- Maintain correct posture in sitting and standing, especially while studying and working on a computer.
- Warm up before engaging in physical activity.
- Keep the spine straight up and down when lifting an object. DO NOT bend over. Use the muscles of your legs and hips to lift.

Exercises for the Lower Back

The following exercises will help to stretch and strengthen your lower back:

- Curl up

- Knee to chest

- Elbow-to-knee stretch

4

- Cat and camel

- Lunge stretch

- Modified chest lift

What Is Poor Body Posture?

You can evaluate your posture by standing in front of a three-panel mirror, of the kind often found in fitting rooms. See Figure 4.1 for guidance on good and poor posture.

Why Have Good Posture?

- Good posture makes your bones align properly
- This bone alignment allows for muscles, joints, and ligaments to work properly
- Internal organs are in the right position and can work more effectively (allows for deep breathing and proper digestion)
- Lessens risk of lower back pain
- Good posture projects the body image that you are strong and proud, not weak and bored

Signs of Poor Posture

- Head aligned in front of center of gravity (can cause headaches, dizziness, and neck, shoulder, and arm pain)
- Too much outward curve in upper back (can shorten breath by squeezing lung area; can cause neck, shoulder, and arm pain)
- Too much inward curve in lower back (can cause low-back pain, painful menstruation)
- Abdomen sticks out too far (can cause **lordosis**, low-back pain, painful menstruation)
- Knees extend backward too much (can cause knee injury and lordosis) **Figure 4.2**

Ways to Improve Your Posture

- **Sit correctly:** Distribute weight evenly on both hips, bend knees at a right angle, legs should not be crossed and feet should be flat on the floor, keep back straight and shoulders back.
- **Stand correctly:** Hold head up with chin in, ears should be in line with shoulders, shoulders should be back, chest forward, knees straight, stomach tucked in.
- **Lift correctly:** Keep back straight and bend at knees and hips, keep feet in wide stance, lift object using leg muscles, moving in a steady motion.
- **Lie in bed correctly:** Lie on your side with your hips and knees slightly bent; put a flat pillow between your knees **Figure 4.3**
.

Figure 4.3

To improve your posture, sleep on your side with your hips and knees slightly bent.

Forward tilt of pelvis

Good Posture   Poor Posture

Figure 4.1

Good posture depends on the pelvic tilt and abdominal muscles. Only when the pelvis is level is it at its strongest.

What's the word. . .

lordosis
Excessive pelvic tilt.

Figure 4.2

Left to right: good posture (pelvic tilt); poor posture (lordotic back, pelvis tilted too far forward; pelvis tilted too far back)

Reflect >>>> Reinforce >>>> Reinvigorate

Knowledge Check

Answers in Appendix D

1. In assessing your flexibility, you should:
   A. Warm up before you do a stretch test.
   B. Do fast moves to get your muscles warm.
   C. Bounce at the end of each movement.
2. What are three basic types of stretching?
   A. Fast, slow, ballistic
   B. Static, ballistic, PNF
   C. Active, passive, quick
3. You can help prevent low-back pain by
   A. Lying flat on your back while sleeping.
   B. Always standing with your legs at least two feet apart.
   C. Exercising your back and abdominal muscles regularly.

Modern Modifications

Think about the activities you do and postures you take each day. Are there ways you can improve your flexibility and posture, just by changing the way you do these activities? When you are sitting or standing, are you

- Arching your back?
- Rounding your shoulders?
- Letting your head slump forward?

When you are lying down, are you

- Tilting your pelvis down?
- Arching your back?

While lying on your back, you should have just enough room between the small of your back and the floor to slide a computer mouse under there. You know your posture is bad if your back is touching the floor (squishing the mouse) or arching (the mouse could do jumping jacks).

Consciously change what you do during each activity or posture. For instance:

- While sitting, keep your back straight, lean slightly forward, and use a footrest to keep your knees higher than your hips.
- While standing, use a footrest to raise one leg to help you keep your back straight.
- When lifting, bend at the knees, NOT at the waist, lift slowly, and push with your legs. Don't twist.
- Do one different stretching exercise each morning, at noon, and each evening before going to bed.

Critical Thinking

Answers in Appendix D

Ready for Fitness?

Scenario One: After standing around waiting for a delayed gun, you bolt from the starting line of a 5K, feeling fit and ready to have a great race. As you sizzle through the first half-mile, you marvel at how fast you are running and how easy the pace feels to you. Suddenly, agonizing pain stabs you, and you are forced to hobble to a complete stop. You realize that you have torn your hamstrings so badly that you probably won't run at anything faster than a very slow jogging pace for at least 6 to 8 weeks.

1. Can stretching before exercising help prevent muscle injuries?
   A. Yes
   B. No
2. Which is the safest type of stretching for most people?
   A. Ballistic
   B. Static
   C. Proprioceptive neuromuscular facilitation (PNF)

Scenario Two: Craig, as a dentist, bends over patients daily for long hours. When he was younger, he experienced no back problems. However, in middle age, he has experienced severe back pain.

3. Does flexibility decrease as a person ages?
   A. Yes
   B. No
4. Could having a "pot belly" affect his flexibility?
   A. Yes
   B. No

Going Above and Beyond

Websites

American Academy of Orthopaedic Surgeons
http://orthoinfo.aaos.org

Georgia State University: Flexibility
http://www.gsu.edu/~wwwfit/flexibility.html

MedlinePlus
http://www.nlm.nih.gov/medlineplus

National Institute on Aging
http://www.n.a.nih.gov/exercisebook

The Physician and Sports Medicine
http://physsportsmed.com

References and Suggested Readings

Canham-Chervak M. et al. Does stretching before exercise prevent lower-limb injury? *Clinical Journal of Sport Medicine 10*(3)(2000): 216.

Gleim G. W. and McHugh M. P. Flexibility and its effect on sports injury and performance. *Sports Medicine 24*(1997): 289–299.

Hodges P. and Jull G. Does strengthening the abdominal muscles prevent low back pain? *Journal of Rheumatology 27*(9)(2000): 2286–2288.

Knudson D. Stretching: from science to practice. *Journal of Physical Education, Recreation and Dance 69*(3)(1998): 38–42.

Knudsen D. V. Stretching during warm-up: do we have enough evidence? *Journal of Physical Education, Recreation and Dance 70*(2)(2000): 271–277.

Patel A. T. and Ogle A. A. Diagnosis and management of acute low back pain. *American Family Physician 61*(6)(2000): 1779–1786

Shrier I. Stretching before exercise: an evidence based approach. *British Journal of Sports Medicine 34*(5)(2000): 324–325.

Shrier I. and Gossal K. Myths and truths of stretching. *Physician and Sports Medicine 28*(8)(2000): 57–63.

CHAPTER 5

Increasing Muscular Strength and Endurance

Objectives

After reading this chapter, you should be able to:

- Explain the difference between muscular strength and muscular endurance, and how training differs for each.
- Describe the changes that take place in your body as a result of muscle training.
- Explain the differences in muscle fibers and their functions.
- Assess muscular strength and endurance.
- Describe effective individual muscle-training exercises.
- Design an effective muscle-training program.

How Strong Are You?

Push-Up Test for Muscular Endurance

- Pick a space on the floor, clear of obstructions.
- Warm up for 3 to 5 minutes before starting.
- Take a couple of minutes to recover after warming up.

For men:

- Take a position with the body straight, toes tucked under, hands about shoulder-width apart and straight under the shoulders (Figure 5.1).
- Lower the body until the elbows reach 90°, or place a paper cup or soft object beneath to touch with your chest.
- Return to starting position with arms fully extended.
- Keep your back straight during the entire push-up.
- Do as many push-ups as you can without stopping.

For women:

- Women tend to have less strength in the upper body and should use the modified push-up position (Figure 5.2).
- Instructions are the same as for men, except that women should perform the test with the knees remaining on the floor.

See (Table 5.1) to rate your fitness level.

Push-up

Figure 5.1

Modified push-up.

Figure 5.2

Table 5.1	Rating Your Fitness by Number of Push-Ups and Modified Push-Ups					
	Number of Push-Ups					
Men	Very Poor	Poor	Fair	Good	Excellent	Superior
Age: 18–29	Below 22	22–28	29–36	37–46	47–61	Above 61
30–39	Below 17	17–23	24–29	30–38	39–51	Above 51
40–49	Below 11	11–17	18–23	24–29	30–39	Above 39
50–59	Below 9	9–12	13–18	19–24	25–38	Above 38
60 and over	Below 6	6–9	10–17	18–22	23–27	Above 27
	Number of Modified Push-Ups					
Women	Very Poor	Poor	Fair	Good	Excellent	Superior
Age: 18–29	Below 17	17–22	23–29	30–35	36–44	Above 44
30–39	Below 11	11–18	19–23	24–30	31–38	Above 38
40–49	Below 6	6–12	13–17	18–23	24–32	Above 32
50–59	Below 6	6–11	12–16	17–20	21–27	Above 27
60 and over	Below 2	2–4	5–11	12–14	15–19	Above 19

Source: Based on norms from the Cooper Institute for Aerobics Research, Dallas, Texas. From *The Aerobics Program for Total Well-Being* by Kenneth H. Cooper, MD, MPH. Copyright© 1982 by Kenneth Cooper. Used with permission of Bantam Books, a division of Random House, Inc.

What's the word...

muscular endurance
The ability of muscles to apply force repeatedly.

muscular strength
The force muscles can exert against resistance.

Muscular Endurance

Muscular endurance describes how long or how many times (number of repetitions) you can lift and lower a given weight. It can be assessed by determining the number of repetitions of a particular exercise that can be performed.

For most people, developing muscular endurance is more important than **muscular strength**. Muscular endurance is usually more important in carrying out everyday activities.

Muscular Strength

As you lift and lower a weight, your muscle must generate enough force to move that weight. Muscle strength can be assessed by determining the amount of weight that can be lifted in one repetition of an exercise. Strength can be developed by increasing the amount of weight that can be lifted in an exercise after a lower weight can be lifted 10–12 times easily.

What Are the Benefits of Muscular Strength and Endurance?

Muscle endurance and muscle strength are important components of physical fitness. Your ability to perform physical tasks can be enhanced by strength and endurance training. The benefits of strength and endurance training are that you will:

- Improve at physical work, sports, and recreation
- Look better and feel better about yourself
- Keep your body weight down more easily
- Better manage stress and anxiety
- Help prevent osteoporosis (brittle-bone disease)
- Have good posture and avoid back and neck pain
- Digest food better (and possibly lower the risk of colon cancer)
- Experience fewer injuries and have better balance

How Does Weight Training Change Body Composition and Metabolism?

Exercising the muscles changes the proportion of fat to muscle fiber and speeds up weight loss. The more muscle, the higher the metabolic rate. It will be easier to keep your weight where you want it by eating right and exercising.

Exercising also slows degeneration of muscle and nerves with age. It keeps the bones strong, helping you to avoid osteoporosis. Being stronger when you are older keeps you from falling down as easily.

Weight training keeps more of your motor nerves connected to the muscles they control. And you are better able to make quick and powerful moves.

Gender Differences for Weight Training

Men are on average larger and stronger than women, because they have more muscle mass. But women have about the same strength in the lower body, and only a small percentage less in the upper body. Why? Men have more androgens (hormones that cause facial hair, deep voice, etc.). Also, male muscles tend to activate faster, adding to muscle power.

What Are the Different Types of Muscle Fiber?

Muscles consist of many muscle fibers. Larger muscle fibers mean a larger and stronger muscle (hypertrophy). When muscle fiber size diminishes it is called atrophy. Two types of muscle fibers exist according to their contraction speed and energy source:

- *Fast-twitch fibers* contract quickly and forcefully, but fatigue more rapidly than slow-twitch fibers. They rely on anaerobic energy metabolism.
- *Slow-twitch fibers* do not contract as rapidly or strongly as fast-twitch fibers. They are fatigue resistant and rely on aerobic energy metabolism.

Endurance activities (i.e., jogging) use slow-twitch fibers; power and strength activities (i.e., sprinting) use fast-twitch fibers. Weight training can increase the size and strength of both of these fiber types.

Everyone has both types of muscle fiber. Your genetics determine which fiber you have most.

Assessing Your Muscular Strength and Endurance

Muscular fitness is determined by assessing muscular strength and endurance.

- Muscular strength: Because muscular strength is specific to the muscle group, the testing of one group of muscles does not provide accurate information about the strength of other muscle groups. For a comprehensive assessment, strength testing must involve several major muscle groups. Standard tests use free weights. The heaviest weight you can lift only one time through the full range of motion for a specific muscle group is considered your maximum strength for that muscle group.
- Muscular endurance: Muscular endurance is specific to each muscle group. Few tests of muscular endurance have been developed. The YMCA developed a bench-press test for muscular endurance, using a standard weight. (Using the bench press to test strength is preferred by some experts. It is not a fair test for smaller, lighter individuals, however.) See Lab 5.1, Activity 1 for complete instructions on how to perform this assessment.

Also see Labs 5.2 and 5.3 for assessing muscular strength and endurance.

Modes of Exercise

Isometric (Static) Exercises

Isometric (static) exercise contracts muscle without changing muscle length (does not involve muscle movement) **Figure 5.3**.

- Do against an immovable object (e.g., a wall) to provide resistance.
- Can be used to strengthen muscles after an injury or surgery.

Advantages

- Requires no or little equipment or expense
- Low risk of muscle soreness
- Can be done in a small space
- Rapid strength improvement

> **The Inside Track**
>
> **Will Weight Training Give Women Bulky Muscles?**
>
> Women do not develop large muscle mass as a result of weight training unless they take steroids and train intensively, as do most female bodybuilders.
>
> The principal advantages of weight training for women are (1) greater strength as they age, (2) better bone density, and (3) easier maintenance of desired weight without fat.

Figure 5.3

Isometric (static) exercise.

Figure 5.4

Isotonic (dynamic) exercise using a weight machine.

Disadvantages

- Difficult to devise a full-body workout
- Not very motivating

Isotonic Exercises

Isotonic (dynamic) exercise contracts muscle in a way that changes muscle length (involves muscle movement). Isotonic is the most popular type of exercise for increasing muscle strength. It can be performed with weight machines **Figure 5.4**, free weights, or your own body (i.e., push-ups). Two kinds of muscle contractions occur **Figure 5.5**:

- *Concentric* occurs when the muscle applies force as it shortens.
- *Eccentric* occurs when the muscle applies force as it lengthens.

For example, during an arm curl, the biceps muscle works concentrically as the weight is raised toward the shoulder, and eccentrically as the weight is lowered.

Advantages

- Improves strength across entire range of motion
- Helps improve joint flexibility
- More motivating

Disadvantages

- Requires more exercise equipment
- Higher risk of muscle soreness

Figure 5.5

Your muscles shorten during concentric action (A), and lengthen during eccentric action (B).

Isokinetic Exercises

Isokinetic exercise combines the advantages of both isometric and isotonic. It uses special apparatus to provide a maximum resistance to the muscles, as in isometric, but throughout the full range of motion, as in isotonic. This equipment is often used by individuals who are in rehabilitation   **Figure 5.6** .

Plyometric Exercises

Plyometrics is doing abrupt, explosive movements, such as bounding on and off a box, or jumping off a platform and immediately leaping upward. This develops quick-twitch muscle fibers, but is risky for injury. Do plyometric exercises only after you have developed well-conditioned muscles.

Figure 5.6

Isokinetic exercise apparatus. *Source:* Image provided by CSMI, www.csmisolutions.com. All rights reserved.

Getting Started with Weight Training

Warm-Up

Begin with a 5 to 10 minute warm-up. This will:
- Prepare the heart muscle and circulatory system
- Warm the muscles, making them more flexible

To warm up, use low-intensity exercises (biking, stair-climbing, treadmill/jogging). When you begin to sweat, you are warmed up.

During Training

According to the American College of Sports Medicine (1998), strength training should be:
- Progressive
- Rhythmic
- Individualized
- Done at a moderate-to-slow speed
- Involve full range of motion
- Stimulate all of the major muscle groups (arms, shoulders, chest, back, legs)
- Not cause labored breathing

Cool Down

Cool down for 2 to 5 minutes with a mild activity (walking, jogging, or cycling). Stretch *after* exercise—warm muscles stretch farther and are less likely to tear.

5

Where Should You Exercise?

At a Health Club/Gym: Advantages

- Availability of professional supervision and trainers
- Many exercise options, including aerobic options
- Social climate: meet new friends
- Influence of motivated exercisers

At Home: Advantages

- Convenient: no concerns about appearance, travel time, parking, gym hours
- Private: avoids strangers, not intimidating if you feel weak and awkward
- No waiting in line; no noise from loud music and talking
- Cleaner: the germs on the bench and bars are yours
- Less expensive: no monthly payments for health club membership

Fundamentals of Weight Training

> **What's the word...**
>
> **repetition (rep)** A single lifting and lowering of the weight.
>
> **set** Number of reps performed without stopping to rest.
>
> **progressive overloading** Increasing, from one session to another, the amount of weight you lift during a set.
>
> **repetition maximums** The maximum weight you can lift successfully once while using proper form.

- To get stronger, use few **repetitions** with maximum weight. The number of repetitions performed without stopping to rest is called a **set**.
- To gain endurance, use many repetitions and minimum weight.

If you train with weights on consecutive days, work the upper body one day and the lower body the next day.

Muscles need one day of rest between training sessions to recover and minimize injury.

Training Frequency

The ACSM (1998) recommends specific training frequencies for various levels of ability:

Beginning: Train entire body 2 to 3 days per week.

Intermediate: Train entire body 2 to 3 days per week.

Split workout: Train each muscle group (upper and lower body) 1 to 2 days per week.

Advanced: Train 4 to 6 days per week.

Elite bodybuilding: Work out twice each day for 4 to 5 days per week—with appropriate steps taken to optimize muscle recovery and minimize risk of overtraining.

Intensity

Intensity is the most critical part of resistance or weight training. It is the amount of weight used in each repetition.

Progressive Overloading

The basis of strength training is **progressive overloading**. This increases the force your muscles can generate, and helps you gain muscle strength without injury.

Progressive overloading has the effect of strengthening individual muscle fibers, and also engaging a larger proportion of available fibers in an activity. This makes you stronger.

If you can lift a certain weight for more than 12 reps with good form, you can increase the weight during your next training session.

Tipping Point

Determining Your Repetition Maximum

- Adjust exercise intensity by knowing your **repetition maximums (RM)**. Use free weights to determine your RMs for various muscle groups.

Creating a Successful Training Program

Start a training routine consisting of one to two sets of 12 reps each for each major muscle group **Figure 5.7** . This takes about 30 minutes to perform. Do this routine two to three times per week.

- Change the exercises you perform for each muscle group every 4 to 8 weeks, even if you keep the same set and rep routine. Changing exercises will overload the muscles differently, increase your strength gains, and alleviate boredom.
- Gradually increase the weight you lift until you can lift it only 12 times with good form. If you can perform more reps easily, increase the weight.
- If you can't do 12 with good form, decrease the weight.
- Increase the weight by no more than 10% per week.
- See Lab 5.3 for tools for tracking your muscular training.

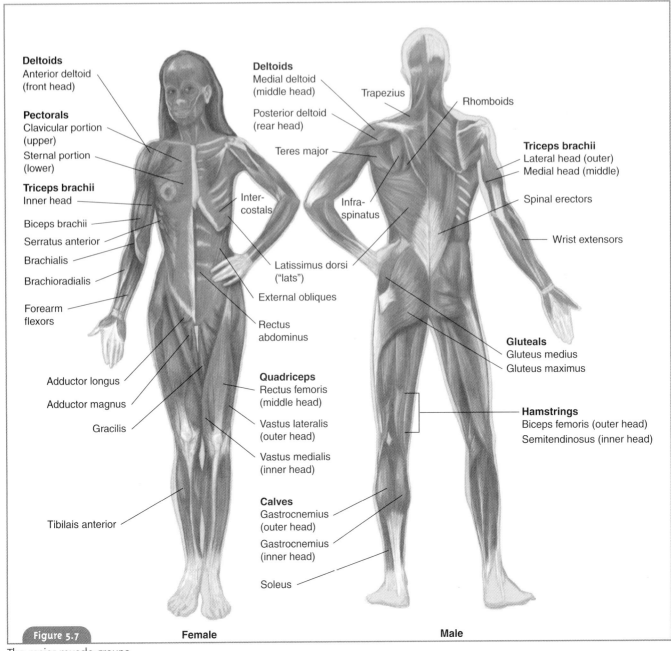

Figure 5.7   **Female**   **Male**

The major muscle groups.

5

Exercise Guidelines

For muscle strength: Three to five sets, two to eight reps, with a weight that cannot be lifted more than eight times.

- Rest at least 120 seconds between sets.
- **DO NOT** perform maximum-weight lifts when strength training.

For muscle endurance: Two to three sets, 12 to 15 reps, with a weight that cannot be lifted more than 15 times.

- Rest 30 to 60 seconds between sets.

Selecting Types of Exercise

Muscle balance refers to the strength ratio of opposing muscle groups across a common joint (e.g., the bicep and tricep muscle groups in the upper arm).

Perform exercises that target opposing muscle groups across joints. You will improve joint function and reduce risk of injury.

Select at least one exercise for each major muscle group.

Exercise Sequence

The ACSM (1998) recommends the following order for exercises:

- Do large muscle group exercises before doing small muscle group exercises.
- Do **multiple-joint exercises** (e.g., squats) before doing single-joint exercises (e.g., leg curl). Why? Because single-joint exercises fatigue the smaller muscle groups needed to perform multi-joint exercises.

An example of a multi-joint exercise is the bench press, because your upper and lower arms move at the shoulder and elbow joints.

An example of a single-joint exercise is a biceps curl because only your lower arm moves at the elbow.

To determine which exercises are multi-joint exercises, watch and feel how many joints move while you perform the exercise.

Lower back and abdominal exercises should be done at the end of your workout because these muscles are used during other exercises for balance and posture. If they are fatigued before doing other exercises, you may not be able to do those exercises properly.

Use Lab 5-3 to help you design your workout and to record your progress.

What's the word...
multiple-joint exercise An exercise in which two or more joints move together.

Weight-Machine Training Safety

- Keep away from moving weight stacks.
- Stay away from moving parts of the machine that could pinch your skin.
- Do not lift in an awkward position.
- Beware of broken bolts, frayed cables, broken chains, or loose cushions.
- Be alert to what is happening around you.
- Be aware of the advantages and disadvantages of using weight machines **Table 5.2** .

Table 5.2	Advantages and Disadvantages of Weight Machines
Advantages	**Disadvantages**
■ Recommended for beginners ■ Convenient ■ Safe: weight cannot fall on you ■ Less clutter: no weights scattered around ■ No spotters needed ■ No lifter needed to balance bar ■ Offer variable resistance ■ Ensure correct lifting movements, which prevents cheating when tired ■ Easy to use: requires less skill than free weights ■ Easy to move from one exercise to the next ■ Easier to adjust ■ Easier to isolate specific muscle groups ■ Back support (on most machines) ■ Some offer high-tech options like varying resistance during lifting motion	■ Limited availability: may need to go to a club ■ Expensive ■ Require a lot of space ■ Do not allow natural movements ■ Most machines have only one exercise ■ Less motivation: only working against resistance on a machine

Weight Machines: Circuit Training

Circuit training combines aerobic and strength exercise.

■ Each exercise station takes 30 to 45 seconds to do.

■ Stations alternate between upper and lower body exercises.

■ The circuit is repeated two or more times per session.

■ Do a circuit-training workout three times a week for aerobic conditioning and moderate increases in strength.

Using Free Weights (Barbells, Dumbbells)

Olympic style barbells with a narrow center bar for gripping and wider ends for loading weights are the most common in gyms.

■ Bar is 5 to 7 feet long and weighs 30 to 45 pounds.

■ Bell plates used to load the bars come in pounds and kilograms. They range from 2.5 to 45 lbs/1.25 to 20 kg.

■ Know if your gym uses plates in pounds or kilograms. 10 lbs is much heavier than 10 kg. Use adjustable collars to keep plates on the bar.

■ Depending on the style of collar, a pair of bells can add 1 to 5 lbs to your bar.

■ Be aware of the advantages and disadvantages of using free weights   Table 5.3 .

5

Table 5.3	Advantages and Disadvantages of Free Weights
Advantages	**Disadvantages**
<ul><li>Allow dynamic movements</li><li>Allow a greater variety of exercises</li><li>Widely available</li><li>Require minimal space</li><li>Strength transfers to daily activities</li><li>Inexpensive</li><li>Offer greater sense of accomplishment</li><li>Most serious bodybuilders and lifters use free weights</li></ul>	<ul><li>Not as safe as exercise machines: weights can fall off the end of the bar or can pin or smash you when muscles tire</li><li>Balancing required, which can be difficult and dangerous (e.g., weights overhead or while doing squats)</li><li>Require spotters for some exercises</li><li>Allow cheating by swinging for momentum when muscles tire</li><li>Require more time to change weights</li><li>Can cause blisters and calluses</li><li>Clutter creates hazard when weights are scattered</li></ul>

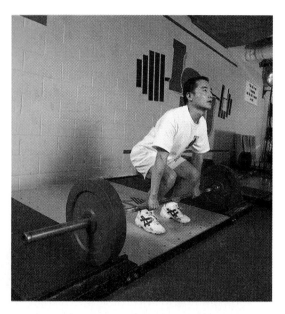

Proper Free-Weight Lifting Techniques

- Keep weights as close to your body as possible.
- Do most of the lifting with your legs.
- Keep your hips and buttocks tucked in.
- Keep your hands dry.
- Wear gloves to prevent calluses and blisters.
- Wrap your thumbs around the bar when gripping it.
- When picking up a weight from the ground, keep your back straight and your head level or up.
- Warm up before lifting.
- Use **spotters** and **collars** with free weights.
- Start slowly and progress gradually.
- Perform exercises smoothly and with good form.
- Lift or push the weight forcefully during the active phase of the lift and then lower it slowly with control.
- Perform all lifts through the full range of motion to reduce the chance of injury and soreness. Do not lock (fully straighten) your knees or elbows when involved in an exercise. This stresses the joint.
- Exhale when exerting the greatest force, and inhale when moving the weight into position for the active phase of the lift.
- Rest between sets if you perform more than one set of each exercise.
- If you feel pain during an exercise, stop immediately. Continue only if the pain subsides, but reduce the amount of weight.
- Soreness the next day is normal when first starting to exercise or when increasing the amount of weight you lift.
- Cool down after a workout.

What's the word. . .

spotter Another person who can help if the weight tilts or can help move a weight into position before or after a lift.

collars Devices used to secure weights to a barbell or dumbbell. Without collars the weights on one side of the bar will slip off.

Improper Free-Weight Lifting Techniques

Do not do the following:

- Bend at the waist with legs straight
- Twist your body while lifting
- Jerk weights; lift smoothly and slowly
- Bounce weights against your body during an exercise
- Arch your back when lifting a weight
- Lift beyond the limits of your strength
- Hold your breath when lifting

Training with Weights

These exercises may be done with free weights or with circuit-training machines.

Bench Press

Muscles developed: pectoralis major, triceps, deltoids. See **Figure 5.8**.

Figure 5.8
Bench press.

- Lie facing up on a bench, your feet flat on the floor, with your head, shoulders, and buttocks pressed down firmly.
- Grip the bar about shoulder width or slightly wider. Push the bar from a low point on your chest to a high point over your chin.
- Extend your arms, pause momentarily, then lower them slowly. Repeat.
- **DO NOT** arch your back or raise your buttocks during lifting.
- **DO NOT** bounce the bar off of your chest.

Shoulder Press

Muscles developed: deltoids, triceps, trapezius. See **Figure 5.9**.

- Stand or sit with your feet shoulder-width apart. Keep your eyes straight ahead and your back straight. Place your hands shoulder-width apart. Push the bar overhead to arm's length, pause, then slowly lower it. Repeat.

Biceps Curl

Muscles developed: biceps, brachialis. See **Figure 5.10**.

- Stand with your feet spread shoulder-width apart, palms facing out. In the starting position, the bar should rest against your thighs. Keep your elbows by your sides, bend your arms slowly to raise the weight up to your chest, pause, then slowly lower it. Repeat.

Triceps Curl

Muscles developed: triceps. See **Figure 5.11**.

- Sit erect with your elbows and palms facing up, the bar resting behind your neck on your shoulders. Your hands should be shoulder-width apart. Slowly curl the weight overhead, pause, and slowly lower it. Repeat.

5

Figure 5.9

Standing military press.

Figure 5.10

Two-arm curl.

Half Squat

Muscles developed: quadriceps, gluteus maximus, hamstrings, gastrocnemius. See Figure 5.12.

- Stand erect with the bar resting on your trapezius muscles (shoulder muscles), not your neck.
- Use an overhand grip, with your hands and feet spread shoulder-width part.
- Lower your weight by bending at the knees to a 90° angle (thighs parallel to floor), pause, and slowly return to an upright position. Repeat.

Figure 5.11

Triceps curl.

Figure 5.12

Half squat.

- Keep your back straight; do not bend forward at the waist.
- **DO NOT** squat beyond halfway or bounce at the bottom.
- Place bench behind you so that you can sit down if you lose your balance. Use spotters.

Heel Raise

Muscles developed: gastrocnemius, soleus. See **Figure 5.13** .

- Stand erect with your hands and feet spread shoulder-width apart.
- Hold the bar resting on your shoulders (see half-squat) or hold a dumbbell in each hand. Use overhand grip.
- With your feet flat on the floor, slowly push down on your toes while lifting your heels as high as possible, pause momentarily, then lower slowly. Repeat.
- You can also do this exercise by placing the front one third of each foot on the edge of a bottom stair or wood block, with the backs of your feet hanging off.

Upright Rowing

Muscles developed: trapezius, deltoids, biceps. See **Figure 5.14** .

- In a standing position, grip bar with palms down 4–8 inches apart.
- Keep your eyes straight ahead and chest high.
- Raise the bar until it reaches chin height, pause momentarily, then lower slowly. Repeat.
- Keep your weight close to the front of your body, and make sure that your elbows stay higher than your hands.

Figure 5.13

Heel raise.

Figure 5.14

Upright rowing.

Figure 5.15

Lunge.

Lunge

Muscles developed: thigh, gluteal. See   Figure 5.15 .

- Place the barbell behind your head or use a dumbbell in each hand.
- Keep the weight of a bar mainly on your trapezius muscles, not your neck.
- Your hands should be shoulder-width apart.
- Keep your head up and look forward, with your back straight.
- Slowly take a step forward and allow leading leg to drop so that it is nearly parallel with floor. Lower part of leg should be nearly vertical and back should be kept upright.
- Pause momentarily, then take a stride with other leg to return to standing position.
- Repeat with other leg.

Training Without Weights

Push-Ups

Push-ups develop triceps, deltoids, pectoralis major, abdominals, and erector spinae   Figure 5.16 .

- Keep your back as straight as possible. Flex elbows. Lower your body until it almost touches the floor; pause momentarily, then raise yourself back up to starting position and repeat.
- You can use a bench, chair, or stairway to support your hands, rather than the floor.
- Increase resistance by having someone push down on your way up.
- If you are unable to do push-ups as described, do modified push-ups by placing your lower body on your knees rather than on your feet   Figure 5.17 .

Figure 5.16

Push-up.

Figure 5.17

Modified push-up.

Figure 5.18

Modified dip.

Figure 5.19

Pull-up or chin-up.

Modified Dip

The modified dip develops triceps, deltoids, and pectoralis major (**Figure 5.18**).

- Place hands on opposite chairs or use parallel bars.
- With knees slightly bent, dip down to at least a 90° angle at the elbow joint, pause momentarily, then raise yourself back up to starting position. Repeat. Increase resistance by having someone push down on your way up.

Pull-Ups and Chin-Ups

Pull-ups and chin-ups develop biceps, triceps, trapezius, and latissimus dorsi (**Figure 5.19**).

- Suspend yourself by your hands and arms from a bar.
- *Pull-ups:* Use overhand grip, palms away, to develop triceps.
- *Chin-ups:* Use underhand grip, palms facing you, to develop biceps.
- Pull body up until chin is above the bar, pause momentarily, then lower yourself to starting position. Repeat.

If you are unable to do a pull-up this way, use a lower bar with your feet on the floor, or have a spotter help by pushing upward at the waist, hips, or legs during the exercise.

Arm Curl

Arm curls develop biceps (**Figure 5.20**).

- Use palms-up grip to raise a bucket filled with rocks, sand, or dirt.
- Start with one arm completely extended. Curl up your arm as far as possible, pause momentarily, then extend arm back to starting position and repeat.
- Repeat exercise with the other arm.

Figure 5.20

Arm curl.

5

Figure 5.21

Curl-up.

Curl-Ups or Crunches

Curl-ups or crunches develop abdominals and hip flexors
Figure 5.21 .

- Lie face up on the floor or an exercise pad, with knees bent at 90° and both feet flat on the floor.
- Fold arms across chest or place hands over your ears—do not lock your fingers behind your head.
- Slowly raise your upper torso into a curling motion until your shoulders have totally cleared the floor.
- Pause momentarily, then slowly return to starting position. Repeat.

Twisting Curl-Up

- Perform the crunch (preceding section), but as you raise your shoulders off of the floor, twist your upper torso to bring your left shoulder toward your right knee.
- Slowly lower yourself back to the starting position.
- Repeat by doing each twist to an alternate side, or alternate sides from one rep to another.

Cautions About Supplements and Drugs

Many people take drugs and supplements to enhance the results of their weight training. This practice can be expensive and dangerous. The most common are anabolic steroids, synthetic derivatives of testosterone. Using this drug helps women bodybuilders develop the muscle mass of men—along with some undesirable secondary sexual characteristics.

Steroids increase protein synthesis, which promotes muscle growth and improves the ability of muscle to respond to training and recovery.

But steroids can also have bad side effects:

- Acne
- Liver and heart damage
- Stunted growth in adolescents
- Females more masculine (body hair)
- Males more feminine (breast development)
- Mood changes (so-called "steroid rage")
- Joint injuries

Other Drugs with Undesirable Side Effects

- *Testosterone* has the same benefits and similar side effects as steroids.
- *Human growth hormone (HGH)* promotes muscle growth, but can cause gigantism: abnormal enlargement of joints, jaw, and skull.
- *Amphetamines* increase motor activity and delay fatigue, but can cause chest pains, extreme confusion, aggressiveness, irritability, and hallucinations.
- *Creatine* is said to increase performance in brief, high-intensity exercises such as sprinting. Side effects include diarrhea, dehydration, and muscle cramping and tearing.
- *Caffeine* also increases motor activity and delays fatigue, but can cause insomnia and abnormal heart rhythm.
- *Androstenedione dehydroepiandrosterone (Andro-DHEA)* promotes muscle growth. It has similar side effects as steroids.
- *Erythropoetin (EPO)* increases red blood cells and the ability to transport oxygen to the muscles. A bad side effect is thickened blood, which can lead to strokes or heart problems.

Reflect ›››› Reinforce ›››› Reinvigorate

Knowledge Check

Answers in Appendix D

1. What is the measure of muscle strength?
   A. Number of repetitions in a set
   B. Length of muscle stretch
   C. Force against resistance
   D. Time taken to complete a workout
2. Which mode of exercise is most popular for increasing strength?
   A. Isometric
   B. Isotonic
   C. Plyometric
   D. Isokinetic
3. What are some of the effects of muscle training on a person's body?
   A. Higher percentage of muscle to fat
   B. Stronger bones
   C. Higher rate of metabolism
   D. All of the above

Modern Modifications

Take a moment to look at your lifestyle in terms of strength training. Would you like to be stronger and more fit? Try these simple suggestions to get started:

- Do a set of push-ups (modified or regular, whichever you are comfortable with) first thing each morning. Only do 1 set of how ever many push-ups you can perform at the moment: 5, 10, 15 whatever that number may be. Every week try adding 1–2 more push-ups to your routine.
- Do a wall squat while you are waiting for class or a meeting to start.
- Take a stress ball to work or class—improve your grip strength and your mood at the same time!
- Grab a can of soup and do some bicep curls while watching television.

Critical Thinking

Answers in Appendix D

Scenario One: As Susan has gotten older her upper arms have become flabby. She is very self-conscious when she raises an arm while wearing short sleeves.

1. What is the reason for lack of firmness in the upper arms?
   A. Untrained muscle
   B. Excess fat
2. Will exercising the upper arms accomplish "spot reduction"?
   A. Yes
   B. No

Scenario Two: Jim was always told that eating several pounds of beef and up to a dozen raw egg yolks daily would bulk up his muscles in addition to lifting weights.

　3. What accounts for large muscles in addition to weight training?

　　A. A high protein diet

　　B. Male hormones

　4. Do most supplements for building muscle mass work?

　　A. Yes

　　B. No

Scenario Three: Phil wants to start a strength-training program. He has been told that exercise machines are better for beginners than free weights.

　5. Why might this be true?

　　A. Widely available

　　B. Less expensive

　　C. Spotters are not needed

Going Above and Beyond

Websites

American College of Sports Medicine

http://www.acsm.org

The National Strength and Conditioning Association

http://www.nsca-cc.org

National Council of Strength and Fitness

http://www.ncsf.org

The Physician and Sports Medicine

http://www.physsportsmed.com

References

American College of Sports Medicine (ACSM). The recommended quantity and quality of exercise for developing and maintaining cardiorespiratory and muscular fitness and flexibility in healthy adults. *Medicine and Science in Sports and Exercise* 30(6)(1998): 975–991.

Braill P. A. et al. Muscular strength and physical function. *Medicine and Science in Sports and Exercise* 32(2)(2000): 412–416.

Ebben W. P. and Jensen R. L. Strength Training for Women. *Physician and Sports Medicine* 26(5)(1998): 86.

Feigenbaum M. S. and Pollock M. L. Strength training: rationale for current guidelines for adult fitness programs. *Physician and Sports Medicine* 25(2)(1997): 44.

_____. Prescription of resistance training for health and disease. *Medicine and Science in Sports and Exercise* 31(1)(1999): 38–45.

Stamford B. Weight training basics. part 1: choosing the best options. *Physician and Sports Medicine* 26(2)(1998): 115–116.

CHAPTER 6

Choosing a Nutritious Diet

Objectives

After reading this chapter, you should be able to:

- Identify the main nutrients and their functions in the body.
- Describe how the body converts nutrients to energy.
- Describe how the body uses energy during exercise.
- List the recommendations of nutrition guidelines and assessments useful in selecting a proper diet.
- Evaluate foods and supplements using their labels.
- Recognize the problems you might encounter in changing your diet and ways to deal with them.

Eating Habits

Calories come from food—all kinds of food. Do you get enough? More than you need? Think about your eating patterns and why you eat what you eat. Check all the answers that describe your eating patterns.

What Do I Usually Eat?

☐ A varied and balanced diet.
☐ A diet with only moderate amounts of fats and sugars.
☐ Deep-fat-fried and breaded foods.
☐ "Extras," such as salad dressings, potato toppings, spreads, sauces, and gravies.
☐ Sweets and rich desserts, such as candies, cakes, and pies.
☐ Snack foods high in fat and sodium, such as chips and other "munchies."
☐ Soft drinks.

When Do I Usually Eat?

☐ At mealtime.
☐ While studying.
☐ While preparing meals or clearing the table.
☐ When spending time with friends.
☐ While watching TV or participating in other activities.
☐ Anytime.

Where Do I Usually Eat?

☐ At home at the kitchen or dining room table.
☐ In the school cafeteria.
☐ In fast-food places.
☐ In front of the TV or while studying.
☐ Wherever I happen to be when I'm hungry.

Why Do I Usually Eat?

☐ It's time to eat.
☐ I'm hungry.
☐ Foods look tempting.
☐ Everyone else is eating.
☐ Food will get thrown away if I don't eat it.
☐ I'm bored or frustrated.

Changes I Want to Make

1. _____

2. _____

3. _____

Source: U.S. Department of Agriculture. *Dietary guidelines and your health: Health educator's guide to nutrition and fitness.* Washington, DC: U.S. Government Printing Office, 1992.

What's the word...

nutrients Substances in food the body needs for normal function and good health.

macronutrients Nutrients needed by your body in relatively large amounts.

micronutrients Nutrients needed by your body in relatively small amounts.

protein Nutrient made up of amino acids that is needed for growth to build, repair, and maintain body tissues.

essential amino acids The nine protein amino acids that the body cannot make, and therefore must come from foods you eat.

complete protein Contains all the essential amino acids.

incomplete protein A protein lacking one or more of the essential amino acids.

What Is a Healthy Diet?

Eating is one of life's greatest pleasures. Since there are many foods and many ways to build a healthy diet and lifestyle, there is plenty of room for choice.

Eating is also a necessity. Nutrients must come from what you eat, because some nutrients cannot be made in the body at all, and others not in sufficient quantities.

The six classes of nutrients are proteins, fats, carbohydrates, vitamins, minerals, and water.

- Proteins, fats, carbohydrates, and water are **macronutrients**.
- Vitamins and minerals are **micronutrients**.

Proteins

All the cells in your body are made up of proteins. Proteins vary in size, depending on how many amino acids are linked together. The proteins are made up of at least twenty different amino acids. Nine are called **essential amino acids** because the body cannot make them; they must be obtained from the diet. That is why you must eat protein—to take in the essential amino acids. Good sources of protein are fish, lean meat, poultry, milk, and beans.

Complete and Incomplete Proteins

Eating protein made up of amino acids is necessary for good health. There are two types of proteins, *complete* and *incomplete*.

Complete proteins are found in animal products (e.g., meats, milk, fish, eggs).

Incomplete proteins generally have one amino acid in insufficient quantity (the limiting amino acid). Grains, legumes, and nuts are sources of incomplete proteins.

How Much Protein Do You Need?

Many people eat high-protein foods because they think that proteins make them grow bigger and stronger.

- Each day adults need about 8 grams for every 20 pounds of body weight (your ideal weight, that is). Athletes may need a bit more.
- You can estimate your protein intake using food labels or by using the Food Guide Pyramid to get an ample amount of protein.

- Taking in a lot of protein increases your fluid needs, and may dehydrate you if you are not taking in enough fluids.
- Eating excessive amounts of protein for a long time requires lots of calcium since some of the calcium may be pulled from the bones. Excessive amounts may contribute to obesity, heart disease, and certain forms of cancer.
- Protein deficiency is the most common form of malnutrition in the world. It can manifest itself in two forms: kwashiorkor and marasmus. Kwashiorkor is distinguished by swelling of body tissues. Marasmus results from chronic protein deficiency and is distinguished by severe **wasting** of body fat and muscles. (Insel, Turner, and Ross 2002)
- Although proteins provide energy, they are not the main source of energy for the body.

Lipids (Fats, Oils)

Lipids (fats) may have a bad reputation, but not all fats are the same.

Benefits of Fat Intake

Fats provide a major form of stored energy; they provide energy during exercise, in cold environments, and when you do not have enough to eat. They:

- Insulate your body
- Cushion internal organs
- Help carry other nutrients throughout your body
- Serve a structural role in making and repairing cells
- Satisfy hunger and add taste to many foods

Cholesterol

Cholesterol is important in forming certain key hormones (e.g., testosterone and estrogen). The body makes cholesterol in the liver. Too much cholesterol in the blood is associated with an increased risk for heart disease. Deposits of cholesterol can build up inside the arteries, which narrow an artery enough to slow or block blood flow.

Cholesterol is carried by **lipoproteins**. When you have your cholesterol checked, the results will show your total blood cholesterol level. If you fasted overnight before giving a blood sample, the test should also show separate counts for your **high-density lipoprotein (HDL)** and **low-density lipoprotein (LDL)**. In general, the higher your LDL and the lower your HDL, the greater your risk for heart disease.

Saturated Fats and Trans Fats: The Bad Fats

Saturated fats are found primarily in animal foods (red meats, butter, poultry with skin, and whole-milk dairy products). Tropical oils such as palm and coconut are also high in saturated fat (Table 6.1).

Taking in too much saturated fat can raise the amount of LDL cholesterol in your bloodstream, increasing your risk of heart disease.

Because saturated fat and cholesterol are not known to help prevent chronic diseases, they are not required in any diet.

Trans fatty acids are unsaturated fats converted (hydrogenated) to a form that has the same bad effects as saturated fats. Trans fats are often found in commercial baked goods, margarines, snack foods, processed foods, and fast foods.

What's the word...

unsaturated fat Type of fat obtained from plant sources and fish; two types are monounsaturated and polyunsaturated.

monounsaturated High concentrations of unsaturated fat in canola, peanut, and olive oils.

polyunsaturated High concentrations of unsaturated fat in sunflower, corn, soybean oils, and fish.

carbohydrates Nutrient that is the body's main source of energy; consists of sugars and starches found in grains, vegetables, and fruits; two types are simple and complex.

glucose Simple sugar circulating in the blood.

glycogen Complex carbohydrates stored primarily in the skeletal muscles and liver. When energy is needed, glycogen is converted to glucose.

Table 6.1	Dietary Fats	
Type of Fat	**Main Sources**	**Effect on Blood Cholesterol Levels**
Monounsaturated	Olives; olive oil, canola oil, peanut oil; cashews, almonds, peanuts, and most other nuts	Lowers LDL; raises HDL
Polyunsaturated	Corn, soybean, safflower oil; fish	Lowers LDL; raises HDL
Saturated	Whole milk, butter, cheese, ice cream; red meat; chocolate; coconuts	Raises both LDL and HDL
Trans fatty acids	Most margarines; vegetable shortening; partially hydrogenated vegetable oil; deep-fried chips; many fast foods; most commercial baked goods	Raises LDL

Food manufacturers hydrogenate foods to improve shelf life. The more processed foods you eat, the greater your trans fat intake. Trans fatty acids are worse for cholesterol levels than saturated fats because they not only raise LDLs but also lower HDLs.

Monounsaturated and Polyunsaturated Fatty Acids: The Good Fats

When unsaturated fats—monounsaturated and polyunsaturated—were eaten in place of carbohydrates, these good fats decreased LDL levels and increased HDL levels, and thus lowered the risk of heart disease.

- Monounsaturated fatty acids are found in olive oil, canola, and peanut oils.
- Polyunsaturated fatty acids are found in fish, sunflower, corn, wheat, nuts, soybean, and vegetable oils. Fish (e.g., mackerel, salmon, sardines, swordfish) are sources of omega-3 fatty acids, which have the potential to lower heart disease risk. The American Heart Association recommends that everyone eat at least two servings of fish a week.

High-Fat Diet and Your Health

A high-fat diet usually means saturated fat. It is associated with many diseases, including heart disease, cancer, obesity, and diabetes. However, a completely fat-free diet can be harmful, since certain fats are essential nutrients.

Limit the bad fats and replace them with good fats. Try to reduce both the trans and saturated fats as much as possible and replace them with polyunsaturated and monounsaturated fats.

Saturated fats have no nutritional value and nobody knows if you need any at all.

Carbohydrates

Carbohydrates are the main source of energy for your body. Your body breaks down most of them to a simple sugar, glucose, also called "blood sugar." Glucose is the most important source of energy for your body. It is stored in your liver and muscle as glycogen.

There are two types of carbohydrates: simple and complex.

- Examples of foods containing simple carbohydrates are table sugar, honey, fruit, milk, maple syrup, and molasses.
- Examples of foods containing complex carbohydrates are whole grains, fruits, vegetables, and legumes (peas and beans).

Complex carbohydrates consist of starch (digestible) and fiber (indigestible). For health reasons you should take in a sufficient amount of fiber every day.

Glycemic Index

The glycemic index measures how different foods affect your blood sugar levels
　Table 6.2　. For example, white bread and potatoes cause blood sugar to rise rapidly. Therefore, they are classified as having a high glycemic index. Apples and brown rice are

Table 6.2	Glycemic Index

Cereals

All Bran	51
Bran Buds + psyll	45
Bran Flakes	74
Cheerios	74
Corn Chex	83
Cornflakes	83
Cream of Wheat	66
Frosted Flakes	55
Grapenuts	67
Life	66
Muesli, natural	54
Nutri-grain	66
Oatmeal, old fach	48
Puffed Wheat	67
Raisin Bran	73
Rice Chex	89
Shredded Wheat	67
Special K	54
Total	76

Fruit

Apple	38
Apricots	57
Banana	56
Cantalope	65
Cherries	22
Dates	103
Grapefruit	25
Grapes	46
Kiwi	52
Mango	55
Orange	43
Papaya	58
Peach	42
Pear	58
Pineapple	66
Plums	39
Prunes	15
Raisins	64
Watermelon	72

Snacks

Chocolate bar	49
Corn chips	72
Croissant	67
Doughnut	76
Graham crackers	74
Jelly beans	80
Life Savers	70
Oatmeal cookie	57
Pizza, cheese & tomato sauce	60
Pizza Hut, supreme	33
Popcorn, light microwave	55
Potato chips	56
Pound cake	54
Power bars	58
Pretzels	83
Saltine crackers	74
Shortbread cookies	64
Snickers bar	41
Strawberry jam	51
Vanilla wafers	77
Wheat Thins	67

Crackers

Graham	74
Rice cakes	80
Rye	68
Soda	72
Wheat Thins	67

Cereal grains

Barley	25
Basmati white rice	58
Bulgar	48
Couscous	65
Cornmeal	68
Millet	71

Sugars

Fructose	22
Honey	62
Maltose	105
Table sugar	64

Pasta

Cheese tortellini	50
Fettucini	32
Linguini	50
Macaroni	46
Spaghetti, 5 min. boiled	33
Spaghetti, 15 min. boiled	44
Spaghetti, protein rich	28
Vermicelli	35

Soups/vegetables

Beets, canned	64
Black bean soup	64
Carrots, fresh, boiled	49
Corn, sweet	56
Green pea, soup	66
Green pea, frozen	47
Lima beans, frozen	32
Parsnips	97
Peas, fresh, boiled	48
Split pea soup w/ ham	66
Tomato soup	38

Drinks

Apple juice	40
Colas	65
Gatorade	78
Grapefruit juice	48
Orange juice	46
Pineapple juice	46

Milk products

Chocolate milk	35
Custard	43
Ice cream, vanilla	60
Ice milk, vanilla	50
Skim milk	32
Soy milk	31
Tofu frozen dessert	115
Whole milk	30
Yogurt, fruit	36
Yogurt, plain	14

Beans

Baked	44
Black beans, boiled	30
Butter, boiled	33
Cannellini beans	31
Garbanzo, boiled	34
Kidney, boiled	29
Kidney, canned	52
Lentils, green, brown	30
Lima, boiled	32
Navy beans	38
Pinto, boiled	39
Red lentils, boiled	27
Soy, boiled	16

Breads

Bagel, plain	72
baquette, French	95
Croissant	67
Dark rye	76
Hamburger bun	61
Muffin, apple cinnamon	44
Muffin, blueberry	59
Muffin, oat & raisin	54
Pita	57
Pizza, cheese	60
Pumpernickel	49
Sourdough	54
Rye	64
White	70
Wheat	68

Root crops

French fries	75
Potato, new, boiled	59
Potato, red, baked	93
Potato, sweet	52
Potato, white, boiled	63
Potato, white, mashed	70
Yam	54

Table 6.3	Sample Substitutions for High-Glycemic-Index Foods		
High-Glycemic-Index Food	Low-Glycemic-Index Alternative	High-Glycemic-Index Food	Low-Glycemic-Index Alternative
Bread, wheat	Oat bran, rye, or pumpernickel bread	Plain cookies and crackers	Cookies made with dried fruits and whole grains such as oats
Processed breakfast cereal	Unrefined cereal such as oats (either museli or oatmeal)	Cakes and muffins	Cakes and muffins made with fruit, oats, or whole grains
Bananas	Apples	Potatoes	Pasta or legumes

Source: Insel, P., Turner, R. E., Ross, D. *Nutrition, 2nd ed.* Sudbury, MA: Jones and Bartlett Publishers, 2004, 149.

digested slower and cause a lower and more gradual change in blood sugar, and therefore, have a lower glycemic index (Table 6.3).

Both diabetes and heart disease have been associated with high glycemic index foods. Type 2 diabetes can be helped by lower glycemic indexed foods.

It is wise to eat minimally processed whole-grain products rather than highly processed grains, cereals, and sugars.

Main Uses of Carbohydrates in Your Body

Your body uses carbohydrates as:

- Fuel in the form of glucose, the most important source of energy in our body. Glucose is stored in the liver and muscle as glycogen. The complex carbohydrates you eat are digested into simple sugars, mostly glucose, and then used by the muscles, brain, heart, and other organs for energy.
- building blocks to make chemicals needed by the cells in the body
- chemical cement for repairing structures of the body

Fiber

There are two categories of **dietary fiber**: soluble and insoluble. **Insoluble fiber** binds with water to help produce bowel movements. Good sources of insoluble fiber are wheat products, leafy vegetables, and fruits (Table 6.4). **Soluble fiber** is associated with reduced levels of cholesterol. Good sources of soluble fiber include oatmeal and beans. Evidence suggests that fiber in your diet may help in the following ways:

- Fiber in wheat bran and oat bran is effective in relieving and preventing constipation.
- Insoluble fiber can lower the risk of diverticular disease.
- A diet high in fiber is linked to a lower risk of type 2 diabetes.

Table 6.4	Foods Rich in Soluble and Insoluble Dietary Fiber		
Rich in Soluble Fiber	**Rich in Insoluble Fiber**	**Rich in Soluble Fiber**	**Rich in Insoluble Fiber**
Fruits		**Nuts and seeds**	
Apples	Apples	Peanuts	Almonds
Cranberries	Bananas	Pecans	Sesame seeds
Grapefruit	Berries	Walnuts	Sunflower seeds
Mango	Cherries	**Legumes**	
Oranges	Pears	Most legumes	Most legumes
Vegetables		**Grains**	
Asparagus	Broccoli	Oat bran	Brown rice
Broccoli	Green peppers	Oatmeal	Whole-wheat breads
Brussels sprouts	Red cabbage	Psyllium	Wheat-bran cereals
Carrots	Spinach		
	Sprouts		

Source: Adapted from Shils M. E., Olson J.A., Shike M., Ross A. C., eds. *Modern Nutrition in Health and Disease,* 9th ed. Philadelphia: Lippincott Williams & Wilkins, 1999.

- A high fiber intake, especially those found in grains, has been linked to a lower risk of heart disease.
- Fiber in your diet promotes weight control by enhancing a full feeling.

Despite what many people think, large studies have not found a link between fiber and a reduced risk for colon cancer.

The recommended daily intake for total fiber per day is 20–35 grams.

Vitamins

You must get vitamins from food and a daily multiple vitamin because your body cannot make them. In the body, vitamins:

- Release energy from carbohydrates, lipids, and proteins
- Help grow and repair tissue
- Maintain and support reproductive functions
- Produce the immune response

Types of Vitamins

Fat-soluble vitamins dissolve in fat, can be stored in the body, and are not excreted in the urine. They include four vitamins: A, D, E, and K.

Water-soluble vitamins dissolve in water and cannot be stored by the body in significant amounts. They include vitamin C and eight B vitamins: thiamin (B_1), riboflavin (B_2), niacin (B_3), pyhridoxine (B_6), cobalamin (B_{12}), folate, pantothenic acid, and biotin. Excess amounts are excreted in the urine.

Vitamin Excesses and Deficiencies

A healthy, balanced diet provides most of the vitamins your body needs. Taking large doses of vitamin supplements can (if fat-soluble) result in an accumulation in the body excessive enough to cause you harm. On the other hand, not getting enough of the right kinds of vitamins in your diet can cause health problems as well   Table 6.5   .

What's the word...

vitamin Nutrient necessary for normal functioning of the body; two types are water-soluble and fat-soluble.

6

Table 6.5 — Major Vitamins

Vitamin	Major Functions	Rich Food Sources	Deficiency Signs/Symptoms	Toxicity Signs/Symptoms
A and provitamin A (beta carotene)	Vision in dim light, growth, reproduction, maintains immune system and skin, antioxidant	Liver, milk, dark green and leafy vegetables; carrot, sweet potato, mango, oatmeal, broccoli, apricot, peaches, and romaine lettuce	Poor vision in dim light, dry skin, blindness, poor growth, respiratory infections	Intestinal upset, liver damage, hair loss, headache, birth defects, death (beta-carotene is less toxic than A)
D	Bone and tooth development and growth	Few good food sources other than fortified milk and eggs	Weak, deformed bones (rickets)	Growth failure, loss of appetite, weight loss, death
E	Antioxidant: protects cell membranes	Vegetable oils, whole grains, wheat germ, sunflower seeds, almonds	Anemia (rarely occurs)	Intestinal upset, bleeding problems
C	Scar formation and maintenance, immune system functioning, antioxidant	Citrus fruits, berries, potatoes, broccoli, peppers, cabbage, tomatoes, fortified fruit drinks	Frequent infections, bleeding gums, bruises, poor wound healing, depression (scurvy)	Diarrhea, nosebleeds, headache, weakness, kidney stones, excess iron absorption and storage
Thiamin	Energy metabolism	Pork, liver, nuts, dried beans and peas, whole-grain and enriched breads and cereals	Heart failure, mental confusion, depression, paralysis (beriberi)	No toxicity has been reported
Riboflavin	Energy metabolism	Milk and yogurt, eggs and poultry, meat, liver, whole-grain and enriched breads and cereals	Enlarged, purple tongue; fatigue; oily skin; cracks in the corners of the mouth	No toxicity has been reported
Niacin	Energy metabolism	Protein-rich foods, peanut butter, whole-grain and enriched breads and cereals	Skin rash, diarrhea, weakness, dementia, death (pellagra)	Painful skin flushing, intestinal upset, liver damage
Vitamin B_6	Protein and fat metabolism	Liver, oatmeal, bananas, meat, fish, poultry, whole grains, fortified cereals	Anemia, skin rash, irritability, elevated homocysteine levels	Weakness, depression, permanent nerve damage
Folate (folic acid)	DNA production	Leafy vegetables, oranges, nuts, liver, enriched breads and cereals	Anemia, depression, spina bifida in developing embryo, elevated homocysteine levels	Hides signs of B_{12} deficiency; may cause allergic response
B_{12}	DNA production	Animal products	Pernicious anemia, fatigue, paralysis, elevated homocysteine levels	No toxicity has been reported

Source: Alters, S., Schiff, W. *Essential Concepts of Healthy Living*, 3rd ed. Sudbury, MA: Jones and Bartlett Publishers, 2003, 212.

Daily Multivitamin Supplement

Walter Willet (2001) with the Harvard School of Public Health says that most people in the United States get enough vitamins to prevent the classic deficiency diseases. He also states that although we may prevent the classic deficiency diseases, most of us do not get enough of five key vitamins that may be associated in preventing several chronic diseases. These vitamins include:

- Folic acid
- Vitamin B$_6$
- Vitamin B$_{12}$
- Vitamin D (see **Figure 6.1**)
- Vitamin E

A standard, store-brand, RDA-level multivitamin can supply you with enough of these vitamins. Such a supplement cannot replace healthy eating, but it is an inexpensive way of providing a nutritional safety net. See **Table 6.6** for newly recognized findings on vitamins.

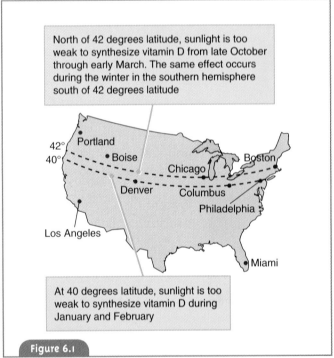

North of 42 degrees latitude, sunlight is too weak to synthesize vitamin D from late October through early March. The same effect occurs during the winter in the southern hemisphere south of 42 degrees latitude

At 40 degrees latitude, sunlight is too weak to synthesize vitamin D during January and February

Figure 6.1

Mapping vitamin D synthesis. Vitamin D synthesis halts for part of the winter if sunlight is too weak. In Los Angeles and Miami, the sunlight is strong enough to synthesize vitamin D year round, even in January.

Table 6.6	Newly Recognized Findings on Vitamins	
Vitamin	**New or Suspected Roles in Health and Disease**	**Daily Optimal Intake**
A	Stimulates production and activity of white blood cells, takes part in remodeling bone, helps maintain health of endothelial cells (those lining the body's interior surfaces), regulates cell growth and division	5000 IU for men; 4000 IU for women
B$_6$	May help fight heart disease and some types of cancer	1.3 to 1.7 milligrams
B$_{12}$	May help fight heart disease and some types of cancer; may help those with dementia or Alzheimer's disease	6 micrograms
Folic acid	Reduces chances of mothers having children with birth defects (spina bifida or anencephaly); may help fight heart disease and some types of cancer	400 micrograms
C	Controls infections; neutralizes harmful free radicals; helps make collagen, which is needed for healthy bones, teeth, gums, and blood vessels	90 mg for men; 75 mg for women (add extra 35 mg for smokers); as evidence unfolds, 200 to 300 mg
D	Helps body absorb and retain calcium and phosphorus, both critical for building bone; keeps cancer cells from growing and dividing; prevents risk of fractures; low intake increases risks of prostate, breast, colon, and other cancers	5 micrograms up to age 50; 10 micrograms between ages 51 and 70; 15 micrograms after age 70
E	Thought to prevent heart attacks, further studies are needed	15 milligrams from food or 22 IU from natural-source or 33 IUs of synthetic form; may need 400 IU or more for optimal health
K	Helps make 6 of the 13 proteins needed for blood clotting; involved in building bone; reduces risk of hip fracture	80 micrograms for men; 65 micrograms for women

Source: Adapted from Willett W. C. *Eat, Drink, and Be Healthy.* New York: Fireside, 2001.

6

Minerals

Minerals are essential for a variety of important bodily functions. (They regulate fluid balance, conduct nerve impulses, and contract muscles) Table 6.7 .

Minerals are classified according to the body's needs: At least 16 **macrominerals** are essential to health (e.g., sodium, chloride, potassium, calcium, phosphorus, magnesium).

Microminerals are **trace minerals** (e.g., iron, zinc, copper, manganese, molybdenum, selenium, iodine, and fluoride).

Two of the most important minerals for keeping yourself healthy are calcium and iron. Calcium is especially important for women, to ward off **osteoporosis** in later life. Iron is important for women to prevent **anemia**.

Water

Water in the body serves many important purposes:

- Excrete wastes
- Maintain blood circulation throughout the body
- Maintain body temperature
- Digest and absorb nutrients

Table 6.7	**Some Essential Minerals**			
Mineral	Roles	Rich Food Sources	Deficiency Signs/ Symptoms	Toxicity Signs/ Symptoms
Calcium	Builds and maintains bones and teeth, regulates muscle and nerve function, regulates blood pressure and blood clotting	Milk products; fortified orange juice, tofu, and soy milk; fish with edible small bones such as sardines and salmon; brocooli; hard water	Poor bone growth, weak bones, muscle spasms, convulsions	Kidney stones, calcium deposits in organs, mineral imbalances
Potassium	Maintains fluid balance, necessary for nerve function	Whole grains, fruits, and vegetables, yogurt, milk	Muscular weakness, confusion, death	Heart failure
Sodium	Maintains fluid balance, necessary for nerve function	Salt, soy sauce, luncheon meats, processed cheeses, pickled foods, snack foods, canned and dried soups	Muscle cramping, headache, confusion, coma	Hypertension
Magnesium	Regulation of enzyme activity, necessary for nerve function	Green leafy vegetables, nuts, whole grains, peanut butter	Loss of appetite, muscular weakness, convulsions, confusion, death	Rare
Zinc	Component of many enzymes and the hormone insulin, maintains immune function, necessary for sexual maturation and reproduction	Meats, fish, poultry, whole grains, vegetables	Poor growth, failure to mature sexually, improper healing of wounds	Mineral imbalances, gastrointestinal upsets, anemia, heart disease
Selenium	Component of a group of antioxidant enzymes, immune system function	Seafood, liver, and vegetables and grains grown in selenium-rich soil	May increase risk of heart disease and certain cancers	Hair and nail loss
Iron	Oxygen transport involved in the release of energy	Clams, oysters, liver, red meats, and enriched breads and cereals	Fatigue, weakness, iron-deficiency anemia	Iron poisoning, nausea, vomiting, diarrhea, death

Source: Alters, S. and Schiff, W. *Essential Concepts of Healthy Living, 3rd ed.* Sudbury, MA: Jones and Bartlett Publishers, 2003, 214.

Tipping Point

- Drink 8.5 cups of water a day to stay properly hydrated. With all of the coffee and soda we drink it is important to still drink water.

About 60% of your total body weight is water. If you lose even 4% of your body weight through sweat, you'll lose the ability to make decisions, concentrate, or do physical work. If you lose as much as 20%, you will die.

Water is lost:

- From breathing
- From sweating
- In urine and stool

Water is taken in from:

- Water in food (fruits, vegetables, soups, meats, grains)
- Water in beverages (e.g., water itself, fruit juices, milk, sport drinks)
- Metabolism or chemical breakdown of foods

If you lose more water than you take in, you become dehydrated. Dehydration can happen if you are:

- Not drinking enough fluids daily
- Working or exercising in a hot or cold environment
- At high altitudes
- Drinking too much alcohol
- Drinking mostly caffeinated liquids (e.g., coffee, tea, colas)

Clear urine is a sign that you are well hydrated. The more dehydrated you are, the darker (and smellier) your urine will be.

You can restore lost fluids by drinking water. Eating foods high in water content also helps restore fluids (adapted from American College of Sports Medicine position stand).

Before exercise:

- Drink about 16 ounces (2 cups) of fluid about 2 hours before exercise to promote adequate hydration and allow time for excretion of excess water.

During exercise:

- Drink fluids at regular intervals to replace water lost through sweating.
- Drink fluids cooler than ambient temperature (between 60° and 72°F)—they are absorbed better.

During exercise lasting more than one hour:

- A sports drink (contains carbohydrates and/or electrolytes) might be considered when exercising more than 1 hour.
- For exercise lasting less than 1 hour, it does not matter if you are drinking water or a sports drink.

After exercise:

- Consider weighing yourself before and after exercising to determine how much fluid you have lost—for every pound of weight lost, you should drink 16 ounces of fluid (2 cups).
- If you feel thirsty, you are already 1–2% percent dehydrated.

6

Free Radicals and Antioxidants

Normal metabolism creates free radicals. Free radicals can damage cell membranes and mutate genes.

Free radical production is increased by cigarette smoke, exhaust fumes, radiation, too much sunlight, some drugs, and too much stress (**Figure 6.2**).

Antioxidants do battle with free radicals, and undo the damage they cause.

Get your antioxidants by eating a variety of fruits and vegetables. If you take supplements instead:

Figure 6.2

Free radical production is increased by exposure to cigarette smoke, exhaust fumes, and radiation.

- The health benefits of **phytochemicals** come from working in combination (**Table 6.8**).
- Isolated phytochemicals may cause more harm than good if taken in high doses.

Table 6.8	Phytochemicals in Fruits and Vegetables and Their Possible Benefits	
Food	**Phytochemicals**	**Possible Benefits**
Berries blueberries, strawberries, raspberries, blackberries, currants, etc.	Anthocyanides, ellagic acid	antioxidants cancer prevention
Chili Peppers	Capsaicin	possible antioxidant topical pain relief
Citrus Fruits oranges, grapefruit, lemon, limes, etc.	Flavanones (tangeretic, nobiletin, hesperitin) Carotenoids	antioxidants
Cruciferous Vegetables broccoli, kale, cauliflower, brussels sprouts, cabbage, mustard greens	indoles isothiocyanates sulphoraphane carotenoids	antioxidants anti-cancer properties
Garlic Family garlic, onions, shallots, leeks, chives, scallions	Allylic sulfides Flavonoids (quercetin)	anti-cancer properties
Soy	daidzein, equol, genestein, entero-lactone, and other plant estrogens	reduce risk of breast, prostate cancer reduce risk of heart disease

Source: Edlin, G., Golanty, E. *Health and Wellness, 8th ed.* Sudbury, MA: Jones and Bartlett Publishers, 2004, 99.

How Your Body Produces Energy

You need energy to move. When you are doing nothing, your metabolic rate is low. If you start moving, your **metabolism** increases.

How do you get the energy to move around—or run a marathon? You get it from the carbohydrates, fats, and proteins in food.

During digestion, most carbohydrates are converted to glucose. Some glucose remains in the blood, where it can be used as a quick source of energy. The rest of the glucose is converted to glycogen and stored in the liver, muscles, and kidneys. When glycogen stores are full, leftover glucose is converted to body fat ⬤ **Figure 6.3** ⬤.

Protein is used mainly to build tissue. But some protein may also be stored as body fat. When other energy fuels run out, the body uses the protein in body fat for energy.

Your body cells convert glucose, glycogen, and fat to **adenosine triphosphate (ATP)**. When a cell needs energy, it breaks down ATP.

When you exercise, your body mobilizes its stores of fat to increase ATP production. ATP can be used in two ways: with oxygen (**aerobic**) or without oxygen (**anaerobic**).

ATP contracts your muscles during exercise. The amount of ATP needed depends on how long and how hard your body works.

Aerobic and Anaerobic Activity

If a movement is quick, occurring at the beginning of exercise, and at high points of exercise intensity, the body uses the small amount of ATP in the cells (e.g., sprinting; a clean and jerk weight lift).

If the movement must be sustained over time, during prolonged but low to relatively moderate exercise (e.g., jogging or running for a distance), the body must create the supply of ATP.

What's the word...

metabolism The rate at which your body uses energy.

adenosine triphosphate (ATP) The only useable form of energy used in the human body.

aerobic Using oxygen.

anaerobic Without using oxygen.

EXTRACTION OF ENERGY

Protein	Carbohydrates	Fats
(amino acids)	(sugars)	(fatty acids)

Molecular building blocks

Energy

Amino acids &	Glucose &	Fatty acids &
body protein	glycogen	lipids

BIOSYNTHESIS

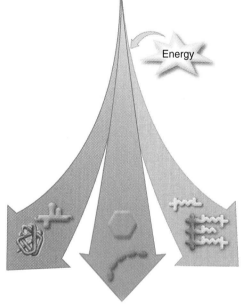

Cells use metabolic reactions to extract energy from food and to form building blocks for biosynthesis.

The Energy Systems

Three different energy systems create energy: immediate energy system, anaerobic energy system, and aerobic energy system. Each system is defined by the way it produces and uses ATP Table 6.9.

Immediate Energy System

ATP is the immediate source of energy within all cells of our body for activities such as sprinting. There are small stores of ATP within skeletal muscle, and these energy stores provide immediate energy to sustain physical activities for a short time. Once the ATP is used, it breaks down into adenosine diphosphate (ADP). For regeneration of ADP into ATP for more energy, creatine phosphate (CP) is needed. It is the CP that regenerates the ATP. Without CP, ATP could provide energy for only a few seconds. With CP, the ATP-CP system can provide energy for about 30 seconds before other energy systems must take over.

Anaerobic Energy System

When vigorous-intensity exercise continues beyond 30 seconds, the only way to continue providing ATP to the exercising muscle is by using glucose in the muscle. Glucose is obtained from glycogen. However, in the process of generating ATP from glucose, lactic acid is formed. Normally, there is only a small amount of lactic acid in the blood and muscle. When lactic acid begins to accumulate in the muscle and then blood, you begin to experience muscular fatigue, unless it is cleared by the body. Lactic acid is cleared from the muscle if the intensity of the exercise is moderate. This happens after a few minutes when the aerobic system, which supplies energy for sustained work, kicks in. If a vigorous effort is sustained, fatigue is inevitable within 3 to 5 minutes.

Aerobic Energy System

The aerobic system provides energy to support long-term steady-state exercise, such as long distance running or swimming. Muscles can use both glucose and fatty acids for energy. These fuel sources can be taken from the circulating blood and from stores within the muscle. Glucose is stored as glycogen and fatty acids are stored as triglycerides in the muscle. When long duration activities are performed at a slow pace more "fat," in the form of fatty acids, is used for energy than muscle glycogen.

Role of Energy Systems in Exercise

During most types of exercise, all three energy systems are involved. When exercise duration increases, a shift occurs from anaerobic energy to aerobic energy Table 6.10.

Fit individuals use more stored fat than those who are less active, so they can exercise longer.

As the intensity and duration of your workout increases, more energy is needed to sustain that level of activity, thus more oxygen is required.

The more physically fit you are, the higher your VO_2max, and the more energy you produce. This increases your ability to exercise at a higher level of intensity and for longer periods.

Being aware of how your body produces and uses energy helps you make the connection between nutrition and exercise.

Table 6.9	Characteristics of the Body's Energy Systems

	ENERGY SYSTEM*		
	Immediate	Nonoxidative	Oxidative
Duration of activity for which system predominates	0–10 seconds	10 seconds–2 minutes	>2 minutes
Intensity of activity for which system predominates	High	High	Low to moderately high
Rate of ATP production	Immediate, very rapid	Rapid	Slower but prolonged
Fuel	Adenosine triphosphate (ATP), creatine phosphate (CP)	Muscle stores of glycogen and glucose	Body stores of glycogen, glucose, fat, and protein
Oxygen used?	No	No	Yes
Sample activities	Weight lifting, picking up a bag of groceries	400-meter run, running up several flights of stairs	1500-meter run, 30 minute walk, standing in line for a long time

*For most activities, all three systems contribute to energy prodcution: the duration and intensity of the activity determine which system predominates.

Source: Adapted from Brooks, G. A., et al. *Exercise Physiology: Human Bioenergetics and its Application*, 3d ed. Mountain View, Calif: Mayfield, 2000, Copyright © 2002 Mayfield Publishing Co. Reproduced with permission of The McGraw-Hill Companies.

Table 6.10	Percentage Contributed by Each Energy System to Overall Energy Needs of Various Activities

Physical Activity	Immediate System (%)	Anerobic System (%)	Aerobic System (%)
Running—100 meters	98	2	—
Running—3 miles	10	20	70
Marathon	—	5	95
Swimming—50 meters	98	2	—
Swimming—400 meters	20	40	40
Swimming—1500 meters	10	20	70

What's the word. . .

immediate energy system System using existing cellular ATP during first 10 seconds of activity.

anaerobic energy system System that creates energy for activities that last less than 5 minutes or have frequent rest periods.

aerobic energy system System that creates energy for activities that last less than 5 minutes or have frequent rest periods.

creatine phosphate (CP) Chemical present in muscles that makes ATP rapidly for thirty seconds worth of exercise. Creatine phosphate is produced in the body from the digestion of meat. It can also be found as a supplement. Research is inconclusive as to its benefits or long-term risks.

lactic acid Chemical formed when muscles must use stored glucose or blood sugar to produce ATP.

Put Your Diet into Action

Is your diet meeting your nutrient needs? Answering this question is not an exact science, but there are useful guidelines available.

Comparison to Dietary Reference Intakes

The National Academies' Institute of Medicine changed the way nutritionists and nutrition scientists evaluate the diets of healthy people by creating the dietary reference intakes (DRIs) Table 6.11 .

The DRI goal was not only to prevent nutritional deficiencies, but also to reduce the risk of chronic diseases such as osteoporosis, cancer, and cardiovascular disease.

Table 6.11 | Dietary Reference Intakes (DRI)

The Food and Nutrition Board of the National Academy of Sciences determines recommended nutrient intakes that apply to healthy individuals. Beginning in 1997, the Food and Nutrition Board (with the involvement of Health Canada) began releasing updated recommendations under a new framework called the Dietary Reference Intakes (DRI). In these revisions, target intake levels for healthy individuals in the U.S. and Canada are listed as either Adequate Intake (AI) levels or Recommended Dietary Allowances (RDA). Also, the DRI values include a set of Tolerable Upper Intake Levels (UL) which are levels of nutrient intake that should not be exceeded due to the potential for adverse effects from excessive consumption.

Dietary Reference Intakes (DRI) for vitamins and minerals

Life stage group	Vitamin A (μg/d)[1]	Vitamin D (μg/d)[2]	Vitamin E (mg/d)[3]	Vitamin K (μg/d)	Thiamin (mg/d)	Riboflavin (mg/d)	Niacin (mg/d)[4]	Pantotenic Acid (mg/d)	Biotin (μg/d)	Vitamin B$_6$ (mg/d)	Folate (μg/d)[5]	Vitamin B$_{12}$ (μg/d)	Vitamin C (mg/d)
Infants													
0–6 mo	400*	5*	4*	2.0*	0.2*	0.3*	2*	1.7*	5*	0.1*	65*	0.4*	40*
7–12 mo	500*	5*	5*	2.5*	0.3*	0.4*	4*	1.8*	6*	0.3*	80*	0.5*	50*
Children													
1–3 y	300	5*	6	30*	0.5	0.5	6	2*	8*	0.5	150	0.9	15
4–8 y	400	5*	7	55*	0.6	0.6	8	3*	12*	0.6	200	1.2	25
Males													
9–13 y	600	5*	11	60*	0.9	0.9	12	4*	20*	1.0	300	1.8	45
14–18 y	900	5*	15	75*	1.2	1.3	16	5*	25*	1.3	400	2.4	75
19–30 y	900	5*	15	120*	1.2	1.3	16	5*	30*	1.3	400	2.4	90
31–50 y	900	5*	15	120*	1.2	1.3	16	5*	30*	1.3	400	2.4	90
51–70 y	900	10*	15	120*	1.2	1.3	16	5*	30*	1.7	400	2.4[7]	90
>70 y	900	15*	15	120*	1.2	1.3	16	5*	30*	1.7	400	2.4[7]	90
Females													
9–13 y	600	5*	11	60*	0.9	0.9	12	4*	20*	1.0	300	1.8	45
14–18 y	700	5*	15	75*	1.0	1.0	14	5*	25*	1.2	400[6]	2.4	65
19–30 y	700	5*	15	90*	1.1	1.1	14	5*	30*	1.3	400[6]	2.4	75
31–50 y	700	5*	15	90*	1.1	1.1	14	5*	30*	1.3	400[6]	2.4	75
51–70 y	700	10*	15	90*	1.1	1.1	14	5*	30*	1.5	400	2.4[7]	75
>70 y	700	15*	15	90*	1.1	1.1	14	5*	30*	1.5	400	2.4[7]	75
Pregnancy													
≤18 y	750	5*	15	75*	1.4	1.4	18	6*	30*	1.9	600	2.6	80
19–30 y	770	5*	15	90*	1.4	1.4	18	6*	30*	1.9	600	2.6	85
31–50 y	770	5*	15	90*	1.4	1.4	18	6*	30*	1.9	600	2.6	85
Lactation													
≤18 y	1,200	5*	19	75*	1.4	1.6	17	7*	35*	2.0	500	2.8	115*
19–30 y	1,300	5*	19	90*	1.4	1.6	17	7*	35*	2.0	500	2.8	120
31–50 y	1,300	5*	19	90*	1.4	1.6	17	7*	35*	2.0	500	2.8	120

This table presents Recommended Dietary Allowances (RDA) and Adequate Intakes (AI). An asterisk (*) indicates AI. RDAs and AIs may both be used as goals for individual intake.

[1] As retinol activity equivalents (RAE).

[2] As cholecalciferol.

[3] As α-tocopherol.

[4] As niacin equivalents (NE).

[5] As dietary folate equivalents (DFE).

[6] In view of evidence linking folate intake with neural-tube defects in the fetus, it is recommended that all women capable of becoming pregnant consume 400 μg of folic acid from supplements or fortified foods in addition to intake of food folate from a varied diet.

[7] Because 10 to 30% of older people may malabsorb food-bound vitamin B$_{12}$, it is advisable for those older than 50 years to meet their RDA mainly by consuming foods fortified with vitamin B$_{12}$ or a supplement containing vitamin B$_{12}$.

Choline (mg/d)	Calcium (mg/d)	Phosphorus (mg/d)	Magnesium (mg/d)	Iron (mg/d)	Zinc (mg/d)	Selenium (µg/d)	Iodine (µg/d)	Copper (µg/d)	Manganese (mg/d)	Fluoride (mg/d)	Chromium (µg/d)	Molybdenum (µg/d)
125*	210*	100*	30*	0.27*	2*	15*	110*	200*	0.003*	0.01*	0.2*	2*
150*	270*	275*	75*	11	3	20*	130*	220*	0.6*	0.5*	5.5*	3*
200*	500*	460	80	7	3	20	90	340	1.2*	0.7*	11*	17
250*	800*	500	130	10	5	30	90	440	1.5*	1*	15*	22
375*	1,300*	1,250	240	8	8	40	120	700	1.9*	2*	25*	34
550*	1,300*	1,250	410	11	11	55	150	890	2.2*	3*	35*	43
550*	1,000*	700	400	8	11	55	150	900	2.3*	4*	35*	45
550*	1,000*	700	420	8	11	55	150	900	2.3*	4*	35*	45
550*	1,200*	700	420	8	11	55	150	900	2.3*	4*	30*	45
550*	1,200*	700	420	8	11	55	150	900	2.3*	4*	30*	45
375*	1,300*	1,250	240	8	8	40	120	700	1.6*	2*	21*	34
400*	1,300*	1,250	360	15	9	55	150	890	1.6*	3*	24*	43
425*	1,000*	700	310	18	8	55	150	900	1.8*	3*	25*	45
425*	1,000*	700	320	18	8	55	150	900	1.8*	3*	25*	45
425*	1,200*	700	320	8	8	55	150	900	1.8*	3*	20*	45
425*	1,200*	700	320	8	8	55	150	900	1.8*	3*	20*	45
450*	1,300*	1,250	400	27	13	60	220	1,000	2.0*	3*	29*	50
450*	1,000*	700	350	27	11	60	220	1,000	2.0*	3*	30*	50
450*	1,000*	700	360	27	11	60	220	1,000	2.0*	3*	30*	50
550*	1,300*	1,250	360	10	14	70	290	1,300	2.6*	3*	44*	50
550*	1,000*	700	310	9	12	70	290	1,300	2.6*	3*	45*	50
550*	1,000*	700	320	9	12	70	290	1,300	2.6*	3*	45*	50

Source: Data compiled from *Dietary Reference Intakes for Calcium, Phosphorus, Magnesium, Vitamin D, and Fluoride.* Washington, DC: National Academy Press, 1997. *Dietary Reference Intakes for Thiamin, Riboflavin, Niacin, Vitamin B$_6$, Folate, Vitamin B$_{12}$, Pantothenic Acid, Biotin, and Choline.* Washington, DC: National Academy Press, 1998. *Dietary Reference Intakes for Vitamin C, Vitamin E, Selenium, and Carotenoids.* Washington, DC: National Academy Press; 2000. *Dietary Reference Intakes for Vitamin A, Vitamin K, Arsenic, Boron, Chromium, Copper, Iron, Manganese, Molybdenum, Nickel, Silicon, Vanadium, and Zinc.* Washington, DC: National Academy Press; 2001. These reports may be accessed via http://nap.edu.

Aim for fitness

Aim for a healthy weight   Be physically active each day

Build a healthy base   **Choose sensibly**

Let the Pyramid guide   Choose a diet that is low in
your food choices   saturated fat and cholesterol
                                 and moderate in total fat

Choose a variety of grains   Choose beverages and foods
daily, especially whole grains   to moderate your intake of sugars

Choose a variety of fruits and   Choose and prepare foods with
vegetables daily   less salt

Keep food safe to eat   If you drink alcoholic beverages,
                                 do so in moderation

Figure 6.4

The 2000 Dietary Guidelines for Americans point the way to good health.
(*Source:* U.S. Department of Agriculture, Agriculture Research Service,
Dietary Guidelines Advisory Committee. (2000). *Nutrition and your health:
Dietary guidelines for Americans, 2000* (5th ed.). Home and Garden Bul-
letin No. 232. Washington, DC.)

Comparison to Dietary Guidelines for Americans

The Dietary Guidelines for Americans offers a general picture of your dietary habits. They
do not identify specific foods to eat. They promote food and lifestyle choices that reduce
risk for chronic disease through three basic messages seen in **Figure 6.4** . In January of
2005 the new dietary guidelines were released, emphasizing a healthy approach to choosing a nutritious diet, maintaining a healthy weight, achieving adequate exercise, and
"keeping food safe" to avoid food-borne illness. Appendix A contains the 2005 Dietary
Guidelines for Americans.

Comparison to the Food Guide Pyramid

The U.S. Department of Agriculture (USDA) developed the Food Guide Pyramid to visu-
ally represent the Dietary Guidelines for Americans. The width shows recommended
quantities of consumption: more foods are recommended in the wide part at the bottom,
less as you go up, and very little in the pointed top **Figure 6.5** .

A panel of experts are revising the USDA's pyramid. Experts believe that the pyramid
contains misinformation that does not point the way to healthy eating. They claim that it
is based on shaky scientific evidence, and it has not changed over the years to reflect the
major advances showing the relationship between diet and health.

A new USDA Food Guide Pyramid will be updated and released in 2005. In fact, it
may not take the shape of a pyramid.

Until the revised USDA Food Guide Pyramid is released, another choice is the
Healthy Eating Pyramid developed by faculty members in the Harvard School of Public

Key

- ○ Fat (naturally occurring and added)
- ▽ Sugars (added)

These symbols show fats, oils and added sugars in foods.

FATS, OILS & SWEETS
Use sparingly

MILK, YOGURT & CHEESE GROUP
2-3 servings

MEAT, POULTRY, FISH, DRY BEANS, EGGS & NUTS GROUP
2-3 servings

VEGETABLE GROUP
3-5 servings

FRUIT GROUP
2-4 servings

BREAD, CEREAL, RICE & PASTA GROUP
6-11 servings

Figure 6.5

The Food Guide Pyramid. The USDA's Food Guide Pyramid is a research-based guidance system that helps consumers put the Dietary Guidelines into action. The pyramid shows how many servings to eat from each food group every day. (*Source:* U.S. Department of Agriculture/U.S. Department of Health and Human Services).

Health. It resembles the USDA's pyramid in shape only, and takes into consideration the most recent research about healthy eating.

Fast Food

Fast foods are quick, reasonably priced, and readily available alternatives to home cooking. While convenient and economical for a busy lifestyle, fast foods are typically high in calories, fat, saturated fat, sugar, and salt **Table 6.12**. In order to maintain a healthy diet, it is necessary to choose fast foods carefully.

In general, people with high blood pressure, diabetes, and heart disease must be very careful in choosing fast food because of the high content of fat, sodium, and sugar.

Many fast-food restaurants have switched from beef tallow or lard to hydrogenated vegetable oils for frying. Some restaurants offer low-calorie choices like salads with low-calorie dressing, low-fat milkshakes, whole-grain buns, lean meats, and grilled chicken.

Fast-Food Recommendations

Choose smaller servings. Consider splitting some items to reduce the amount of calories and fat. Ask for a "doggy bag," or simply leave some food on your plate.

- *Pizza:* Ask for less cheese, and choose low-fat toppings such as onions, mushrooms, green peppers, tomatoes, or other vegetables.
- *Sandwiches:* Choose regular or junior-size lean roast beef, turkey, chicken breast, or lean ham. Extras such as bacon, cheese, or mayonnaise will increase fat and calories. Select whole-grain breads over croissants or biscuits—the latter contain added fat.

Table 6.12 — Partial Composition of Selected Fast-Food Items

Food	Total Calories	Total Fat (grams)	Calories from Fat	Cholesterol (milligrams)	Sodium (milligrams)
Big Mac	560	31	280	85	1070
Burrito Supreme	440	18	170	45	1220
French fries (medium/salted)	370	20	180	00	240
Turkey sub sandwich	273	4	34	19	1391
Fried chicken breast	400	24	220	135	1116
Pizza (slice)	300	14	120	25	610
Caesar salad (no dressing)	240	13	120	25	780
Caesar salad (with dressing)	520	43	390	40	1420
Chocolate shake (medium)	320	7	60	20	230

Source: Edlin, G. and Golanty, E. *Health and Wellness,* 8th ed. Sudbury, MA: Jones and Bartlett Publishers, 2004, 105.

- *Hamburgers:* A single, plain meat patty without cheese and sauces is the best choice. Ask for extra lettuce, tomatoes, and onions. Some restaurants feature hamburgers without buns.
- *Meat, Chicken, and Fish:* Look for items that are roasted, grilled, baked, or broiled. Avoid meats that are breaded or fried. Use small portions of heavy sauces, such as gravy, if at all.
- *Salads:* Dressing, bacon bits, and shredded cheese add fat and calories. Choose lettuce and assorted vegetables for most of your salad. Use low-fat or fat-free salad dressings. Ask for the salad dressing on the side.
- *Desserts:* Choose low-fat frozen yogurt, fruit ices, sorbets, and sherbets. But occasional indulgent desserts can add fun to a carefully selected, well-balanced diet.

Vegetarian Diets

Nutrients that may be lacking in a **vegetarian diet** are protein, vitamin B$_{12}$, vitamin D, riboflavin, calcium, zinc, and iron.

Vegetarians who limit or omit animal products from their diets may need to take supplements (e.g., calcium, vitamin B$_{12}$). The various classifications of vegetarian include **lacto-**, **lacto-ovo-**, and **semi** or **partial vegetarian**.

Vegan diets require careful planning in order to obtain adequate amounts of required nutrients.

Mediterranean Diet

The Mediterranean diet is based on the dietary traditions of the countries surrounding the Mediterranean sea (Crete, Greece, Southern Italy, and North Africa). The people who live there exhibit strikingly lower rates of chronic disease.

The traditional diets of the Mediterranean region are mainly based on the foods from a rich diversity of plant sources, and include fruits, vegetables, whole grains, beans, nuts, and seeds. Fruits and vegetables are locally grown and often consumed raw or processed very little. This may be significant to their potential value for fiber and antioxidants.

- In North Africa, couscous, vegetables, and legumes are the core of the diet.
- In southern Europe, the diet includes rice, polenta, pasta, and potatoes, with vegetables and legumes.

What's the word. . .

vegetarian diet Diet in which vegetables are the foundation and meat products are restricted or eliminated.

vegan Person who eats only foods of plant origin.

lacto-vegetarian Person who includes some or all dairy products in his or her diet.

lacto-ovo-vegetarian Person who includes milk, dairy products, and eggs in his or her diet.

semi or partial vegetarian Person who eats no red meat, but may include chicken or fish, dairy products, and eggs in his or her diet.

- In the eastern Mediterranean, bulgur and rice, together with vegetables and legumes such as chickpeas, are the main part of many meals.
- Throughout the Mediterranean bread is a staple eaten without butter or margarine.

Characteristics of the Mediterranean Diet

Fish, Poultry, and Red Meat Red meat (associated with colon cancer, prostate cancer, and heart disease) is eaten sparingly. Along with poultry, only about 15 ounces a week is consumed. Fish consumption varies from one country to another, but averages to about 5 to 15 ounces a week.

Dairy Products Cheese and yogurt from goats, sheep, buffalo, cows, and camels are traditionally consumed in low to moderate amounts. In the entire region, very little fresh milk is drank. Butter and cream are used only on special occasions. The bacterial cultures of yogurt may contribute to good health.

Wine with Meals Throughout the Mediterranean, wine is consumed in moderation and is usually taken with meals. For men, moderation is two glasses a day, for women one glass a day.

Olive Oil and Total Fat Olive oil, high in monounsaturated fat, is a good source of antioxidants. It is the main source of fat in the Mediterranean. Current research suggests that olive oil may actually increase HDL (good) cholesterol, but has little effect on LDL (bad) cholesterol.

Physical Activity The people of the Mediterranean engage in physical activity in their everyday lives and consider it vital to good health and proper weight.

Other Ethnic Diets

Every ethnic diet has its healthy and unhealthy foods, sauces, and preparation. The guidelines for healthy eating given in this chapter can be applied to any diet.

The suggestions that follow are based on recommendations from the National Institutes of Health and the American Dietetic Association **Table 6.13** .

Challenges Existing for Special Populations

College Students

College students often on the run, eat fast food, and from dining hall or cafeteria lines. The circumstances of college life make it all too easy to eat food that is not very nutritious or to skip meals, especially breakfast. Think about how, what, and when you eat.

- Don't skip breakfast.
- Take your time when you eat.
- Pick the right foods in the dining hall line or at a fast-food restaurant.
- For snacks, eat granola bars, raw veggies, fruit, low-fat cheese, low-fat yogurt, plain popcorn (no butter!), and soup.
- Drink plenty of water.

Table 6.13	Ethnic Diet Recommendations
Good	**Not As Good**
Chinese Steamed, poached, boiled, roasted, barbecued, or lightly stir-fried fresh fish and seafood, skinless chicken, tofu, with mixed vegetables, Chinese greens, steamed rice, steamed spring rolls, soft noodles, with hoisin sauce, oyster sauce, wine sauce, plum sauce, velvet sauce, or hot mustard	Crab Rangoon, crispy duck or chicken, or anything breaded or deep-fried, including fried rice, fried wontons, egg rolls, and fried or crispy noodles
Thai Dishes barbecued, sautéed, broiled, boiled, steamed, braised, or marinated; skewered and grilled meats; with fish sauce, basil sauce, or hot sauces; bean thread noodles; Thai salad	Coconut milk soup; peanut sauce or dishes topped with nuts; crispy noodles; red, green, and yellow curries containing coconut milk
Japanese Dishes boiled or made in boiling broth, steamed, simmered, broiled, or grilled; with mixed rice, steamed rice, or buckwheat, wheat, or rice noodles	Dishes battered and fried or deep-fried; fried pork cutlet, fried tofu
Mexican Fish marinated in lime juice; soft corn or wheat tortillas, burritos, fajitas, enchiladas, soft tacos, tamales filled with beans, vegetables, or lean meats; with refried beans, nonfat or low-fat rice and beans; with salsa, enchilada sauce, or picante sauce; gazpacho, menudo, or black bean soup; fruit or flan	Crispy fried tortillas; fried dishes such as chile rellenos, chimichangas, flautas, or tostadas; nachos and cheese, chili con queso, and other dishes made with cheese or cheese sauce; guacamole, sour cream; refried beans made with lard; fried ice cream
Italian Pasta primavera or pasta, polenta, risotto, or gnocchi; with marinara, red or white wine sauce, red or white clam sauce, light mushroom sauce; dishes grilled or made with tomato-based sauce, broth and wine sauce, or lemon sauce; seafood stew; vegetable, minestrone, or bean soups	Cheese or smoked meats; dishes prepared alfredo, carbonara, fried, creamed, or with cream; veal scallopini; chicken, veal, or eggplant parmigiana; Italian sausage, salami, or prosciutto; buttered garlic bread; cannoli
French Fresh fish, shrimp, scallops, mussels, or skinless chicken, steamed, skewered and broiled or grilled; without sauces; clear soups	Dishes prepared in cream sauce, baked with cream and cheese, or in a pastry crust; drawn butter, hollandaise sauce, or mayonnaise-based sauce
Indian Dishes prepared with curry and roasted in a clay oven or pan-roasted; kabobs; yogurt and cucumber salad, and other yogurt-based dishes and sauces; lentils and basmati rice; baked bread	Any fried or coconut-milk–based dishes; meat in cream sauce; clarified butter; fried breads

---

What's the word. . .

carbo loading Stuffing yourself with complex carbohydrates during the days before an endurance event.

Athletes

Carbo loading builds and maintains stores of glycogen for muscles, which extends endurance and delays fatigue.

If you are an endurance athlete:

- A few days before an event, gradually increase the amount of complex carbohydrates you are eating to about 70% of your total calories.

- At the same time, gradually decrease the amount of workout time.

- Two to four hours before the event, eat a light meal of bagels, pasta, or breads and cereals.
- Afterward, eat a meal with carbs, protein, and fat to help repair and rebuild muscle.

Not all athletes find that carbo loading helps their performance. Test the effects of the carbo-load diet when you not preparing for competition.

There is no need to take in extra protein; the average American already takes in 50% more calories than needed. As an athlete, you need only 12% protein in your overall daily intake of calories.

Legal supplements (vitamins, minerals, protein, certain amino acids) don't help.

Women

Because they tend to be smaller than men, women require less protein and fewer calories. Women should concentrate on getting enough of the right nutrients, especially:

- *calcium* to head off osteoporosis, a special aging hazard for women, and
- *iron* to avoid anemia, another special hazard for females who menstruate.

Women can get the nutrients they need from nonfat and low-fat dairy, orange juice, fortified cereal, lean red meat, and green leafy vegetables.

Men

Men are at risk for heart disease, cancer, and later-life weight gain, because they tend to eat more red meat and fewer grains, vegetables, and fruits than recommended. They can get the necessary vitamins, minerals, fiber, and phytochemicals from grains, vegetables, and fruit.

Diabetics

Diabetics must watch their diets very carefully, because they must maintain just the right blood sugar level at all times during the day. If the level falls, they must take immediate remedial action, such as drinking orange juice, to bring the level up.

Diabetics must take a blood sugar measurement several times during a day, and new instruments that make it easier to do this are now available.

A diabetic diet should be low in simple sugars, high in foods with a high glycemic index, and include a reasonable amount of nonsaturated fats.

Older People

People over 50 are usually less active, so they need fewer calories to balance the calorie outgo.

The absorption of nutrients in the older digestive tract is less than it was when younger, so it is a good idea to eat foods fortified with vitamin B_{12}, or to take vitamin B_{12} supplements.

Older folks should also make sure they include foods high in fiber in their diet, because regularity is more of a problem.

6

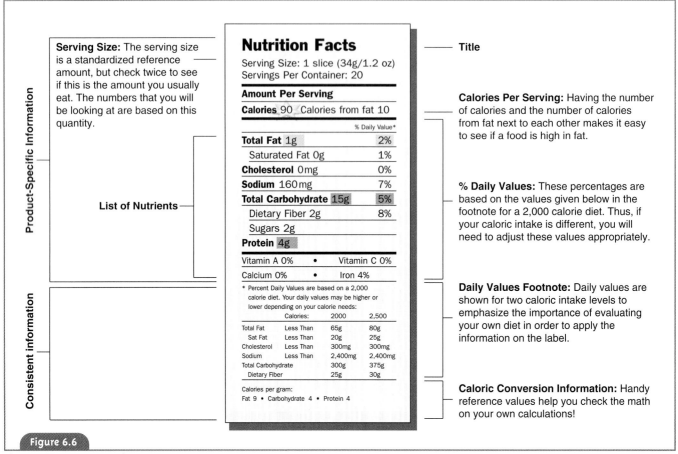

Serving Size: The serving size is a standardized reference amount, but check twice to see if this is the amount you usually eat. The numbers that you will be looking at are based on this quantity.

Product-Specific Information

List of Nutrients

Consistent information

Nutrition Facts
Serving Size: 1 slice (34g/1.2 oz)
Servings Per Container: 20

Amount Per Serving

Calories 90   Calories from fat 10

% Daily Value*

Total Fat 1g	2%
Saturated Fat 0g	1%
Cholesterol 0mg	0%
Sodium 160mg	7%
Total Carbohydrate 15g	5%
Dietary Fiber 2g	8%
Sugars 2g	
Protein 4g	

Vitamin A 0%	•	Vitamin C 0%
Calcium 0%	•	Iron 4%

* Percent Daily Values are based on a 2,000 calorie diet. Your daily values may be higher or lower depending on your calorie needs:

	Calories:	2000	2,500
Total Fat	Less Than	65g	80g
Sat Fat	Less Than	20g	25g
Cholesterol	Less Than	300mg	300mg
Sodium	Less Than	2,400mg	2,400mg
Total Carbohydrate		300g	375g
Dietary Fiber		25g	30g

Calories per gram:
Fat 9 • Carbohydrate 4 • Protein 4

Title

Calories Per Serving: Having the number of calories and the number of calories from fat next to each other makes it easy to see if a food is high in fat.

% Daily Values: These percentages are based on the values given below in the footnote for a 2,000 calorie diet. Thus, if your caloric intake is different, you will need to adjust these values appropriately.

Daily Values Footnote: Daily values are shown for two caloric intake levels to emphasize the importance of evaluating your own diet in order to apply the information on the label.

Caloric Conversion Information: Handy reference values help you check the math on your own calculations!

Figure 6.6

The Nutrition Facts panel.

Smart Food Choices

Looking at Labels

On a food label's Nutrition Facts panel, manufacturers are required to provide information on certain nutrients in a certain order **Figure 6.6** :

- If a claim is made about any of the optional components, or if a food is fortified or enriched with any of them, nutrition information for these components is mandatory.
- The required nutrients address today's health concerns. The order in which the information must appear is the priority of current dietary recommendations.

Dietary Supplement Labels

Supplement labels are limited by law in what they can and cannot say **Figure 6.7** . They:

- Identify the supplement
- Give the quantity (e.g., 40 capsules)
- Give directions for using and storing
- Show warnings, if needed
- List standardization levels, in some cases
- List an address for more information

① "When you need to perform your best, take ginseng." This statement has not been evaluated by the Food and Drug Administration. This product is not intended to diagnose, treat, cure, or prevent disease.

Supplement Facts

Serving Size 1 Capsule

Amount Per Capsule

Oriental Ginseng, powdered (root)   250 mcg*

*Daily value not established

⑥ Other ingredients: Gelatin, water, and glycerin

ABC Company
Anywhere, MD 00001

① Structure/function claim

② Manufacturer's suggested serving size

③ Botanical supplements must list part of plant present and common name (Latin name if common name not listed in "Herbs of Commerce")

④ Information listed per "serving"

⑤ Conventional food nutrients, if present, must be listed

⑥ "Other" dietary ingredients and quantities listed here, if present. For proprietary blends total weight only may be listed, with components listed in descending order of predominance by weight

Figure 6.7
Dietary supplement label.

They are also required to include a "supplement facts" box or panel, showing:

- Serving size
- Source and amount of ingredients assigned daily values
- Name, source, and amount of ingredients not having daily values

By law, supplements can make only three types of claims:

- *Structure-Function* claims (e.g., "Specially formulated to make you feel on top of the world!") are not reviewed by the FDA, so must carry a disclaimer: "This statement has not been evaluated by the Food and Drug Administration. This product is not intended to diagnose, treat, cure, or prevent any disease."
- *Nutrient content* claims must mean the same as they do on food labels. "High potency" may be applied only to single-ingredient supplements with 100% of the daily value, and only to a multi-ingredient supplement if it has a minimum of two thirds of the combined daily values.
- *Disease* claims may be made only if authorized by the FDA or some other such body. A calcium supplement is allowed to say that it will help prevent osteoporosis, for example.

Food Additives

Additives—mainly sugar, salt, and corn syrup, along with citric acid, baking soda, vegetable colors, mustard, and pepper—are added to food to:

- Enhance taste or change appearance
- Help process the food
- Keep the food fresh
- Boost nutritional value

Possible health problems from consuming food with additives include:

- Spells of sweating and a rise in blood pressure for some people after eating food with monosodium glutamate (MSG), used as a flavor enhancer
- Possibly increased (but still low) risk of certain cancers from additives butylated hydroxyanisole (BHA) and butylated hydroxytoluene (BHT) used to keep foods fresh. The FDA is reviewing the use of these additives, and some manufacturers have stopped using them.
- A (usually low) risk of cancer-causing agents in the stomach from consuming the small amounts of nitrates and nitrites added to protect meats from botulism.
- Severe reactions in some people to sulfites used to keep vegetables from turning brown. The FDA strictly limits the use of sulfites and requires such foods to be clearly labeled.

If you are sensitive to an additive. check food labels when you shop and ask questions when you eat out.

Food-borne Illness

What's the word...

pathogens Microorganisms causing disease.

It might surprise you to know this, but **pathogens** causing food-borne illness (commonly called "food poisoning") are more of a threat than additives or pesticide in food.

How can this happen? Try eating undercooked chicken or hamburger, raw ground beef (called *steak tartar* when you do it on purpose), or raw oysters, and you may well find out.

How do you know you have food poisoning? You might mistake it for the flu, with symptoms such as fever, vomiting, diarrhea, and feeling generally weak. You will likely recover, but children and the elderly can further suffer blood poisoning, kidney failure, rheumatic disease, seizures, or death.

Causes

The specific pathogens and associated foods causing food-borne illness include:

- *Campylobacter jejuni* in meat and poultry
- *Cryptosporidium* in drinking water
- *Cyclospora* on fruit
- *E coli* (*Escherichia coli*) in water and meat
- Hepatitis A virus on fruit
- *Listeria monocytogenes* in lunch meat, sausage, and hot dogs
- *Salmonella* in or on eggs, vegetables, poultry
- *Vibrio* in shellfish

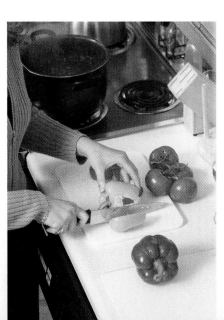

Prevention

Treat your food and your kitchen right, and they will treat you right:

- Put perishable items in the refrigerator right away.
- Do not leave cooked or refrigerated food at room temperature for more than 2 hours.
- Store eggs in the coldest part of the fridge (not the freezer) for no longer than 3–5 weeks.
- Use or freeze fresh poultry, fish, and ground meat within 1–2 days.
- Use or freeze fresh meat within 3–5 days.
- Do NOT thaw frozen food on the kitchen counter. Put it in the regular part of the fridge or use the defrost setting on the microwave.
- Wash your hands before and after you handle food.
- Wash counters, cutting boards, dishes, and utensils before and after handling.

- Use one cutting board for meat and another for foods eaten raw, such as fruits and vegetables.
- Rinse and scrub fruits and vegetables with a brush, then peel.
- Don't eat raw sprouts, or stick them in boiling water for 10 seconds.
- Cook all food sufficiently well.
- Don't put raw eggs in Caesar salad, hollandaise sauce, or eggnog.
- Drink only pasteurized milk and juice.
- Don't leave leftovers in the fridge longer than 3–5 days.
- When in doubt, throw it out.

Treatment

If, in spite of all of these precautions, you think you may have been hit with a food-borne illness:

- Drink plenty of clear fluids to stave off dehydration.
- Rest to recover faster.
- Wash your hands often—always before handling food.

If you have a fever higher than 102°F, blood in the stool, or you are dehydrated, call your doctor or go to the campus clinic, especially if you are sick for more than 2–3 days. Symptoms of botulism are dizziness, vomiting, double vision, and paralysis. If you are experiencing any of them, call 9-1-1 immediately.

Irradiated Foods

Irradiation has been used for a long time to sterilize plastic wrap, milk cartons, teething rings, contact lenses, and medical supplies.

Newer methods of irradiation using electricity and X rays do not require radioactive materials.

Since 1963, the federal government has allowed, one food group at a time, the irradiation of:

- Pork
- Raw poultry
- Red meat
- Fruits
- Vegetables
- Wheat and flour
- White potatoes
- Herbs and spices

All primary irradiated foods have the radura symbol **Figure 6.8** and a brief information label. Irradiation kills most pathogens, but does not completely sterilize. Proper handling is still necessary.

Not many irradiated foods are available, because consumers are skeptical or fearful of them. But when consumers have information about irradiation and its benefits, most want to purchase them.

> **What's the word. . .**
>
> **botulism** Poisoning by the toxin of the microorganism *Clostridium botulinum*.
>
> **irradiation** Treatment with gamma rays, X rays, or high-voltage electrons to kill pathogens and, in the case of food, to increase shelf life.

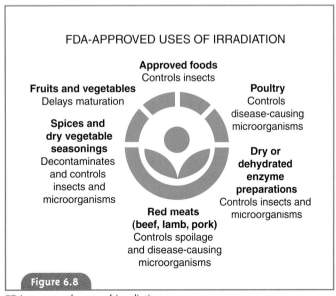

Figure 6.8

FDA-approved uses of irradiation.

FDA-APPROVED USES OF IRRADIATION

Approved foods — Controls insects

Fruits and vegetables — Delays maturation

Poultry — Controls disease-causing microorganisms

Spices and dry vegetable seasonings — Decontaminates and controls insects and microorganisms

Dry or dehydrated enzyme preparations — Controls insects and microorganisms

Red meats (beef, lamb, pork) — Controls spoilage and disease-causing microorganisms

Genetically Modified Foods

How do you modify an organism genetically? You insert genes from one organism into another to introduce new traits or enhance existing ones. Why would you do this? Well, for one thing, it makes crops:

- more resistant to disease, heat, and frost;
- last longer;
- better tasting and more nutritious; and
- requires less fertilizer and pesticides.

This process could save billions in costs, because such crops are more productive. This would help feed the hungry in third world countries.

What is the downside? We don't know if genetic modification of food crops will:

- Create previously unknown "transgenic" organisms that might have adverse effects on us and our environment
- Cross-pollinate and destroy other plants
- Create superweeds that resist herbicides

Whether you know it or not, you have been eating genetically modified foods since 1996, if what you eat comes from a supermarket. So far, such modification seems to be benign and helpful. Only time will tell.

Organic Foods

Concerned about Frankenfood? Don't want to eat meat from cattle fed on growth hormone, or vegetables and fruit sprayed with so many pesticides that even bugs won't eat them? Look for the USDA label . Foodstuffs can't carry it unless:

- Crops meet strict limits on pesticide spraying
- No sewage sludge is mixed into the soil
- Cattle are allowed outdoors and fed only organic feed
- No antibiotics or growth hormones are used
- No genetic engineering or ionizing radiation takes place

There are degrees of organic, however, so check the small print:

- "100% organic" means all organic ingredients; can carry USDA label.
- "Organic" means 95% organic ingredients; can still carry label.
- "Made with organic ingredients" means 70% organic; no label allowed.

Figure 6.9
USDA organic label.

Assessing and Changing Your Diet

How can you tell whether you are getting the right amounts of the essential nutrients to meet your needs? Complete Lab 6.1 to find out.

Stay on the Healthy Path

Now you know what and how to eat and keep yourself healthy. Help yourself stay on the right path: dust off and apply the self-management skills you learned from Chapter 1.

Use the Food Guide Pyramid and the Dietary Guidelines to help you figure out what is good to eat and what to avoid. Then, follow these tips:

- Cook at home.
- Plan ahead when you shop for food.
- Consume only small amounts of meat.
- Have a few meatless meals each week.

Benefits of Food

If you are thinking you should take supplements to get the vitamins you need, think again. You lose out on other essential nutrients if you eat a diet high in calories, fat, and sodium and think you can make up for it with supplements.

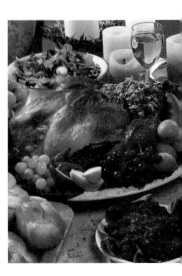

Fruits and vegetables also have much more antioxidants and phytochemicals than supplements:

- Three fourths of a cup of cooked kale (with a lot less of vitamins E and C) will neutralize as many free radicals as approximately 80 times as much vitamin E or more than 50 times as much vitamin C in supplement form.
- Other sources of antioxidants high in oxygen radical absorbance capacity (ORAC) units include blueberries, blackberries, strawberries, prunes, plums, raisins, beets, and red bell peppers—even Brussels sprouts, if you like them.

If you do take supplements, look for the U.S. Pharmacopoeia (USP) symbol on the bottle. The supplement should dissolve completely in under 45 minutes. Supplements that take longer to dissolve won't go into the bloodstream and can't do you any good.

Physical Performance

If physical activity is your thing—especially if you're a competitive athlete—you are always looking for an edge. Our advice? Skip the supplements, and do this:

- Drink enough water.
- Know and consume a well-balanced diet, with enough fruits and vegetables and variety, and you'll get all the vitamins and minerals you need without supplements.
- Skip the protein-rich diet. It is unlikely to build bigger muscles. Worse, it may dehydrate you and take away calcium.
- Include no more than 30% of your total calories in fat.
- Starchy foods high in complex carbohydrates are what your body prefers for fuel.
- Avoid sugary foods. You won't get the same energy boost.

Nutritional Quackery

If you read a typical fitness magazine, you will see no shortage of nutrition advertisements. Popular claims by nutrition quacks (a pretender to medical skill) are that their products and services will:

- Take off body fat and lower weight
- Build muscle
- Boost energy
- Enhance endurance
- Fight fatigue
- Relieve muscle soreness

Dietary Supplements

Just about anything can be sold as long as it is called a "dietary supplement." The FDA considers dietary supplements to be food, so they are not evaluated for safety and effectiveness. People tend to believe that the products on the market have been researched, tested, and inspected.

Avoid buying products with claims like "fat burner," "fat metabolizer," "energy enhancer," "performance booster," "strength booster," "ergogenic aid," "anabolic optimizer," or "genetic optimizer."

How Is Nutritional Quackery Harmful?

- Buying into quackery may increase health risks by preventing you from seeking adequate medical care.
- Products and services by quacks are usually expensive.
- Products and services may detract from scientific nutrition recommendations.
- False claims may promote distrust of the medical community.

Reflect ›››› Reinforce ›››› Reinvigorate

Knowledge Check

Answers in Appendix D

1. The basic form of energy used in the human body is:
   A. GTO
   B. ATP
   C. MAG
   D. TOP
2. The three types of energy systems are:
   A. Short, long, strenuous
   B. Tough, easy, medium
   C. Immediate, anaerobic, aerobic
   D. Carbon dioxide, oxygen, both combined
3. When ordering pizza:
   A. Ask for more cheese.
   B. Refuse extra toppings.
   C. Choose toppings such as green peppers, pineapple, and tomatoes.
   D. Ask for cheese-filled crust.

Modern Modifications

- Try granola bars, raw veggies, fruit, and plain popcorn (no butter) for snacks.
- Drink plenty of water.
- Try to stick with meat dishes that are grilled, baked, roasted, or broiled.
- Have your salad dressing in a separate dish and dip your fork in it before the salad.
- Have sorbet or frozen yogurt instead of ice cream.
- Have a sandwich on whole-grain bread.

Critical Thinking

Answers in Appendix D

Scenario One: Matt is a college student who spends more than an hour a day vigorously exercising.

1. Anyone vigorously exercising over one hour should:
   A. Consider drinking an electrolyte/carbohydrate drink
   B. Drink only water
   C. Feel it is fine to drink soda pop to replace fluids
   D. Tough it out

2. For best absorption of fluids by the body, which temperature is best?

   A. Cooler than ambient temperature

   B. Warmer than ambient temperature

   C. Same as ambient temperature

   D. Temperature does not matter

Scenario Two: Susan lives a very busy life and is on the go most waking hours of the day. Her three children seem to be involved in every sport and activity available through school and community. She exercises daily. She belongs to a book club, volunteers at the local hospital, and is active in her church's programs. She brings home fast-food meals several times a week. She is considering giving vitamin supplements to her family, since she has little time to prepare well-balanced meals at home.

3. Water-soluble vitamins are "safer" than fat-soluble vitamins because excessive amounts are excreted in the urine.

   A. True

   B. False

4. Which is the recommended method for Susan to determine if she needs to give her family a vitamin supplement?

   A. Compare the foods eaten by her family to dietary standards—dietary reference intakes (DRIs).

   B. Have anthropometric measures made.

   C. Obtain a biochemical assessment of body fluids (e.g., blood, urine).

   D. Have a clinical nutrition examination of hair, nails, and skin.

Scenario Three: The popularity of vegetarianism has increased in recent years. Jana has gone vegetarian for several reasons, but mainly because she believes it is healthier.

5. Which vegetarian diet contains no animal products?

   A. Lacto-vegetarian

   B. Lacto-ovo-vegetarian

   C. Vegan

   D. Semi-vegetarian

6. Vegetarians limiting or omitting animal products from their diets may need to take:

   A. Vitamin B_{12}

   B. Calcium supplements

   C. Iron supplements

   D. All the above

Going Above and Beyond

Websites

American Dietetic Association
http://www.eatright.org

Mayo Clinic Diet and Nutrition Resource Center
http://www.mayohealth.org/mayo/common/htm/dietpage.htm

Consumer Information Center: Food
http://www.pueblo.gsa.gov/food.htm

FDA Center for Food Safety and Applied Nutrition
http://vm.cfsan.fda.gov

Gateways to Government Nutrition Information
http://www.nutrition.gov or *http://www.foodsafety.gov*

MedlinePlus: Nutrition
http://www.nlm.nih.gov/medlineplus/nutrition.html

National Cancer Institute 5-A-Day Program
http://www.5aday.gov

USDA Food and Nutrition Information Center
http://www.nal.usda.gov/fnic

Nutrition Analysis Tool, University of Illinois, Urbana/Champaign
http://www.nat.uiuc.edu

Center for Science in the Public Interest
http://cspinet.org

Office of Dietary Supplements
http://dietary_supplements.info.nih.gov
Fast Food Finder
http://www.olen.com/food
Glycemic Index—University of Sydney
http://www.glycemicindex.com

References and Suggested Readings

American Dietetics Association (ADA). Vegetarian diets: position of the American Dietetics Association. *Journal of the American Dietetics Association* 7(1997): 1317–1321.

Clark K. Water, sports drinks, juice, or soda? *ACSM Health and Fitness Journal,* 2(5)(1998): 41.

Foster-Powell et al. International table of glycemic index and glycemic load values: 2002. *American Journal of Clinical Nutrition* 76 2002:5–56.

Insel P., Turner R. E., Ross D. *Discovering Nutrition.* Sudbury, MA: Jones and Bartlett, 2003.

Insel P., Turner R. E., Ross, D. *Nutrition.* Sudbury, MA: Jones and Bartlett, 2002.

Manner M. M. Vitamins and minerals, part I: how much do you need? *ACSM Health and Fitness Journal* 5(1)(2001): 33–36.

Manore M. M. Vitamins and minerals, part II: who needs supplements? *ACSM Health and Fitness Journal* 5(3)(2001): 33–36.

Manore M. M. Vitamins and minerals, part III: can you get too much? *ACSM Health and Fitness Journal* 5(5)(2001): 26–28.

Willet W. C. *Eat, Drink, and Be Healthy.* New York: Fireside, 2001.

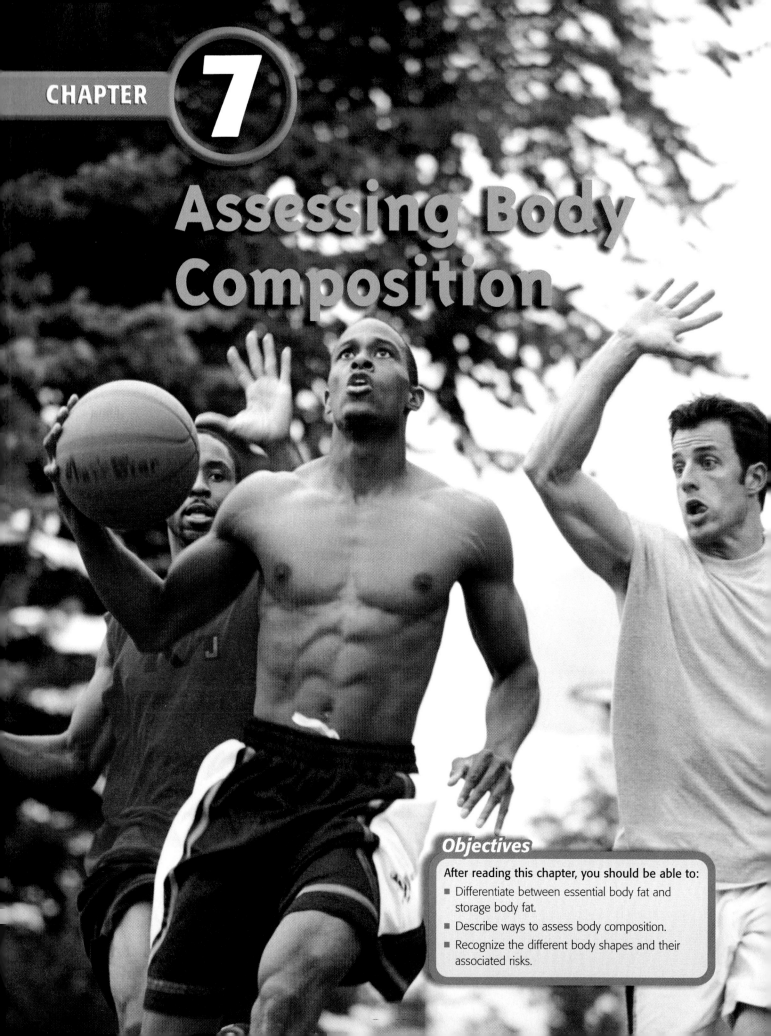

CHAPTER 7

Assessing Body Composition

Objectives

After reading this chapter, you should be able to:

- Differentiate between essential body fat and storage body fat.
- Describe ways to assess body composition.
- Recognize the different body shapes and their associated risks.

A Fast and Easy Way to Find Your Body Composition

Measure Your Waist Circumference

1. Remove your outer clothes from around your waist to make sure the measuring tape is positioned correctly **Figure 7.1** .

2. Place a nonstretchable measuring tape in a horizontal plane around your waist at the tops of your hipbones. (Use a full-length mirror to ensure that the tape is level all around the abdomen.)

3. Make sure the tape is snug without compressing your skin, and parallel to the floor.

4. Breathe out, and then measure.

5. To have a healthy body composition, your waist measurement should be

   - for men, less than 40 inches (102 cm).
   - for women, less than 35 inches (88 cm).

Figure 7.1

What Is Body Composition?

Body composition is more important than overall weight in determining health risks. For example, a person with a ratio of weight to height above some standard may have excess fat (adipose tissue), or may be very fit and muscular and have no weight-related health risk.

Essential Body Fat

Your **essential body fat** resides in your nerve cells, muscles, and bone marrow, as well as in your lungs, heart, liver, and intestines. It has many important functions:

- Keeps your physiological activity normal (e.g., nerve conduction)
- Helps keep your body warm
- Protects your organs from injury
- Stores energy needed when your body is active or when you are injured or ill

The desirable amount of essential fat for a healthy person is:

- Adult women: 10–12% of total body weight
- Adult men: 3–5% of total body weight

Women have more essential body fat in their hips, thighs, breasts, and uterus.

Storage Fat

Some fat beyond what is essential is also desirable. Besides organ protection and body insulation, **storage fat** supplies energy: 3500 calories per pound of adipose tissue **Figure 7.2**.

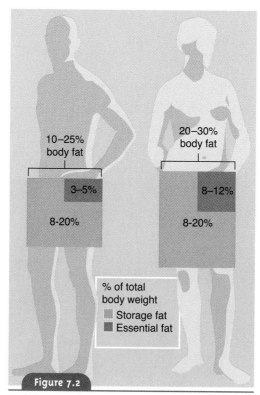

10–25% body fat

3–5%

8-20%

20–30% body fat

8–12%

8-20%

% of total body weight
☐ Storage fat
☐ Essential fat

Figure 7.2

Body fatness of a typical man and woman. (*Source:* Data compiled from Nutrition for physical fitness and athletic performance for adults—Position of ADA and the Canadian Dietetic Association. (1993). *Journal of the American Dietetic Association* 93:691–697. Reprinted with permission from the American Dietetic Association.)

Figure 7.3

Voluptuous women were once considered the female ideal (A); in today's society Jennifer Aniston embodies a popular standard (B).

Determining Recommended Body Composition

Your weight is not necessarily a good indicator of how healthy you are. What is important is the ratio of body fat to lean body mass in your body composition.

For instance, a female bodybuilder may weigh more than a standard chart says she should. But she may have only about 8% to 13% of her body weight in fat. This is probably the least amount of body fat a woman can have and still be healthy.

What society deems as a desirable or ideal body differs in different time periods, usually depending on trends in fashion. It used to be, and still is in some cultures, that women with a good bit of nonessential fat were considered physically attractive and sexually desirable. Today the skinny fashion-model body type is "in" **Figure 7.3** .

Assessing Body Weight

You can assess your body composition by comparing yourself to a weight-to-height table, or by measuring your body mass index.

- Use a scale to measure your weight.
- Use a tape measure to measure your height.

Height–Weight Tables

Many versions of height–weight tables are available, all with different weight ranges. Some tables take into account a person's frame size and age, while others do not.

Body composition measured on a table does not show the proportion of body fat to lean muscle mass. Athletes may be overweight as measured by the table, but not unhealthy.

Too many criticisms exist to recommend the use of height–weight tables.

7

Table 7.1	Classification of BMI Values
BMI	Classification
Below 18.5	Underweight
18.5 to 24.9	Normal
25 to 29.9	Overweight
30 and above	Obese

Body Mass Index

The body mass index (BMI), based on an individual's height and weight, is a helpful indicator of body composition. A BMI number is *not* a certain percentage of body fat.

The BMI can help detect risk of health or nutritional disorders. The BMI number alone is not diagnostic.

A healthy BMI for adults is between 18.5 and 24.9. BMI ranges are based on the effect body weight has on disease and death.

What Does BMI Mean?

You can interpret BMI values for adults with one fixed number, regardless of age or gender, using the guidelines in Table 7.1:

People with a very low or high BMI have a higher relative mortality Figure 7.4.

Figure 7.4
BMI and mortality.

Assessing Body Fatness

Everyone needs a certain amount of fat for stored energy, heat insulation, shock absorption, and other functions. As a rule, women have more fat than men. Experts generally agree that men with more than 25% body fat and women with more than 30% body fat are obese.

The desirable ranges of body fat are:
- Adult women: 20% to 25% of total body weight
- Adult men: 12% to 20% of total body weight

Risk of chronic disease rises when the percent of body fat:
- Exceeds 30% of total body weight in adult women
- Exceeds 25% of total body weight in adult men

Body fatness can be assessed by several methods. Very sophisticated methods such as dual energy X-ray absorptiometry (DEXA), isotope dilution, and CT (computed tomography) and MRI (magnetic resonance imaging) scans more accurately assess body composition; however, their expense may limit their usefulness on a large scale.

Skinfold Measurements

Because half of your body's fat is located under your skin, you can estimate your percentage of body fat by measuring skinfold thickness. This requires some skill.

See Lab 7-1, Activity 4 for complete instructions on how to take a skinfold measurement.

Bioelectrical Impedance Analysis

Body fat percentage can be measured using bioelectrical impedance analysis.
- Electrodes are attached to the wrist and ankle and a small electrical impulse is sent through the body.

What's the word...

body mass index (BMI) A measure of body fatness, calculated by dividing your weight in pounds by your height in inches. Then divide that answer by your height in inches. Multiply the answer by 703.

What's the word...

bioelectrical impedance Measurement of the strength and speed of an electrical signal sent through the body.

- Current flows more easily through the parts of the body composed mostly of water (blood, urine, and muscle) than it does through bone, fat, or air.
- A computer measures the bioelectrical impedance of the signal and combines it with information such as height, weight, and gender to assess percentage of body fat.

Procedure

1. You stand with bare feet on a device resembling a conventional bathroom scale with two built-in footpad electrodes.

   OR

   You lie on a cot and spot electrodes are placed on your hands and bare feet and connected to a bio-electrical impedance machine.

2. A built-in computer measures your bioelectrical impedance, and then uses this number and your gender, height, fitness level, weight, and in some cases your age to assess your percentage of body fat.

Caution

- You need to be adequately hydrated.
- If you are dehydrated, the amount of fat will likely be overestimated.
- People with pacemakers are not candidates for this method.

Disadvantages

- Tends to overestimate your body fat if you are lean and athletic, unless the machine is equipped with an "athlete" mode.
- Does not take into account the location of body fat.

Hydrostatic (Underwater) Weighing

Hydrostatic (underwater) weighing is another method to measure body fat percentage.

Procedure

1. You are weighed while suspended on a trapeze in the air.
2. You are then seated on a special scale and totally submerged in a pool or tank.
3. You exhale as much air as possible and remain motionless as your weight is recorded.
4. The procedure is repeated two to five times to get a dependable weight number.

- Because fat floats, a fat person will weigh less under water than a lean person of the same body weight.
- Your percent of body fat is calculated from equations based on density of body composition.

Bioelectrical impedance.

What's the word...

hydrostatic weighing
Measuring a person's weight while he or she is suspended in water.

Underwater weighing.

Disadvantages

- Underwater weighing requires expensive equipment.
- The procedure requires a well-trained technician.
- The calculation of body fat percentage is based on studies of young Caucasians. The formula may not fit all cases.
- Some people feel uncomfortable when they are fully submerged, leading to incorrect readings.
- There is always air left in the lungs. It is difficult to accurately correct for this.
- It does not take into account the location of body fat.

Bod Pod.

Densitometry (Air Displacement)

Air displacement is more practical to use as a measure of body fat than water displacement. A new device, the Bod Pod, allows an individual to sit in a sealed chamber of known volume and displace a certain volume of air.

Apple shape.

Body Fat Distribution

It is not only how much fat an individual has, but where the fat is on the body that affects a person's health. Women usually collect fat in their hips and buttocks, giving their figures a "pear" shape. Men typically build up fat around their bellies, giving them more of an "apple" shape. This is not a hard and fast rule. Some men are pear-shaped and some women become apple-shaped, especially after menopause. Most people have a combination of both. It's healthier not to develop a beer belly.

Pear shape.

Calculate Your Waist-to-Hip Ratio

Your waist-to-hip ratio (WHR) tells you where you store body fat **Figure 7.5**.

Your WHR = waist circumference (inches) divided by hip circumference (inches).

Standard WHRs for:

- Men should be less than 0.95
- Women should be no more than 0.8

Ratios greater than these indicate a tendency to central (torso) obesity. People who store excess fat centrally, as opposed to in their extremities, are at an increased risk for cardiorespiratory diseases and diabetes.

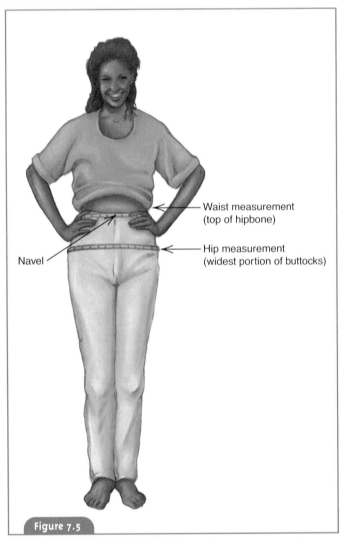

Waist measurement
(top of hipbone)

Hip measurement
(widest portion of buttocks)

Navel

Figure 7.5

To determine one's waist and hip circumferences, measure the
waist directly above the hipbone; measure the hips at the widest
point of the buttocks.

Measure Your Waist Circumference

Some experts believe that measuring your waist is as good as the WHR, and is easier to do.

- See Lab 7-1, Activity 1 for detailed instructions on how to measure your waist circumference.
- Note that if an individual is under 5 feet in height or has a BMI of 35 or above, waist circumference standards used for the general population may not apply.

Importance of Regular Assessment of Body Composition

As most people age, they lose lean body mass, and gain body fat.

From about the age of 25 until 65, most people gain about 40 pounds. They also lose about 20 pounds of lean tissue mass.

That means they have actually gained 60 pounds of fat!

It is important, especially if you are undertaking a weight-loss program of diet and exercise, to reassess your body composition about once a month.

Combine exercise with dieting, because dieting alone can cost you lean body mass. This is not a healthy change in your body composition.

You will be surprised to find that, as a result of the exercise, you have gained more lean mass and lost body fat. If you lost four pounds, you may have gained four pounds of lean mass, meaning you lost eight pounds of fat! Now, isn't that pretty encouraging?

Health Risks of Overweight and Obesity

Overweight is generally defined as a BMI greater than 25 but less than 30, or body fat that is 20–25% for men and 25–30% for women.

Obesity is generally defined as a BMI greater than or equal to 30, or body fat that is more than 25% for men and 30% for women. Both overweight and obesity are discussed in greater detail in Chapter 8.

Reflect ›››› Reinforce ›››› Reinvigorate

Knowledge Check

Answers in Appendix D

1. Body composition consists of:
   A. Fat, muscle, bone, and other body tissues
   B. Storage fat
   C. Essential fat and muscle mass only
2. The risk of chronic disease rises when your body fat:
   A. Is found only in your legs
   B. Exceeds 12% (men) and 20% (women)
   C. Exceeds 25% (men) and 30% (women)
3. You are healthy only if:
   A. You are a bodybuilder whose weight matches your height on a standard chart
   B. Your body shape matches the ideal
   C. You have the right amount of body fat and lean body mass

Modern Modifications

How many times have you vowed to eat better and exercise more? Right. And how long did that effort last? Right again. Is there a way to keep yourself on track to shape up? Yes, there is: Using proven techniques to modify your behavior.

Monitor yourself by observing and recording each aspect of what you do:

- Amount of sedentary time spent per day
- Calories taken in each time you eat something
- The frequency, duration, and intensity of each exercise you do
- Changes in your body shape, composition, and weight as your program progresses

Monitoring is a continuous process of self-motivation. Focus on what matters. Keep records. Use the charts in lab manual to track your progress.

Health Risks of Too Little Body Mass

Dieting Without Exercise

Dieting (or more simply, a change in your eating habits) should be combined with exercise to balance the intake and outgo of calories.

Another major reason to include exercise with dieting or controlled eating is to preserve and build lean body mass, essential for good health. Dieting alone to lose weight often results in unhealthy loss of lean body mass. Weight loss with exercise maximizes the removal of fat, minimizes the loss of protein, and helps maintain the metabolic rate.

It is easier to reduce caloric intake (refusing to eat a piece of cake with 250 calories) than it is to burn off the calories (jogging more than two miles at 110 calories per mile). Dieting alone uses deprivation to achieve weight loss, but with a greater loss of protein (lean tissue) and water. The body becomes less able to burn calories and more fat is eventually gained.

Dieting alone is seldom effective over the long term. Most weight-loss diets fail and the person ends up with more weight and fat than before dieting began.

Reward yourself when you have reached a body change goal. Tangible rewards may include going to a movie you want to see or buying a favorite music CD. Intangible rewards may include taking an afternoon off from work or school.

Numerous small rewards, given to yourself for meeting small goals, are more effective in motivating yourself than bigger rewards that require a longer, more difficult effort.

Critical Thinking

Answers in Appendix D

Scenario One: During Megan's first year in college she gained 12 pounds. Because she didn't like the cafeteria food in her dorm, she ate one or more meals at various fast-food restaurants each day. Moreover, her college did not require a physical education class, so her physical activity involved walking to classes and little else.

1. Which is the most practical method for Megan to assess her *body weight*?
   A. Body mass index (BMI)
   B. Weight-to-height tables
   C. Underwater weighing

2. Which is the most practical method for Megan to assess her *body fat*?
   A. Underwater weighing
   B. Skinfold measurements
   C. Bioelectrical impedance analysis

Scenario Two: Patti has just discovered that her BMI is 27, which means she is considered overweight. She has decided that she will lose the necessary weight to lower her BMI to the healthy score of 23.

3. What is the most effective and healthy way for Patti to lower her BMI score?
   A. exercising 3 times a week without changing her eating habits
   B. going on a strict diet with no exercise
   C. combining regular exercise and a healthy diet

4. How often should Patti be reassessing her body composition?
  A. every 2 weeks
  B. every 3 months
  C. every month

Going Above and Beyond

Websites

American Dietetic Association
http://www.eatright.org

American Obesity Association
http://www.obesity.org

Center for Science in the Public Interest
http://www.cspinet.org

Fast Food Facts: Interactive Food Finder
http://www.olen.com/food

Frontline on Fat
http://www.pbs.org/wgbh/pages/frontline/shows/fat

MedlinePlus on Obesity Weight Loss
http://www.nlm.nih.gov/medlineplus/obesity.html
http://www.nlm.nih.gov/medlineplus/weightlossdieting.html

National Association of Anorexia Nervosa and Associated Disorders (ANAD)
http://www.anad.org

National Eating Disorders Association
http://www.nationaleatingdisorders.org

Office of Dietary Supplements
http://dietary_supplements.info.nih.gov

Shape Up America!
http://shapeup.org

USDA Food and Nutrition Information Center
http://www.nal.usda.gov/fnic
Weight Control Information Network
http://www.pueblo.gsa.gov/cic_text/health/weightloss4life/wtloss.htm
Weightloss2000
http://www.weightloss2000.com

References and Suggested Readings

ACSM. Position stand: appropriate intervention strategies for weight loss and prevention of weight regain for adults. *Medicine and Science in Sports and Exercise* 33(12):2145–2156.

ADA. Weight management: position of the American Dietetics Association. *Journal of the American Dietetics Association* 97(1997):71–74.

Anderson R. E. Exercise, active lifestyle, and obesity: making an exercise prescription work. *Physician and Sports Medicine* 27(10)(1999):41–50.

Foreyt J. P. An etiological approach to obesity. *Hospital Practice,* August 15, 1997: 123–148.

Insel P., Turner R. E., and Ross D. *Discovering Nutrition.* Sudbury, MA: Jones and Bartlett Publishers, 2003:268–270.

_____. *Nutrition.* Sudbury, MA: Jones and Bartlett Publishers, 2002:296–302.

Klem M. L., et al. A descriptive study of individuals successful at long-term maintenance of substantial weight loss. *American Journal of Clinical Nutrition* 66(1997):239–249.

Rubinstein S. and Caballero B. Is Miss America an undernourished role model? *Journal of the American Medical Association* 283(12)(2000):1569.

Wickelgren, I. Obesity: how big a problem? *Science* 280(1998):1364–1376.

CHAPTER 8

Maintaining a Healthy Body Composition and Body Weight

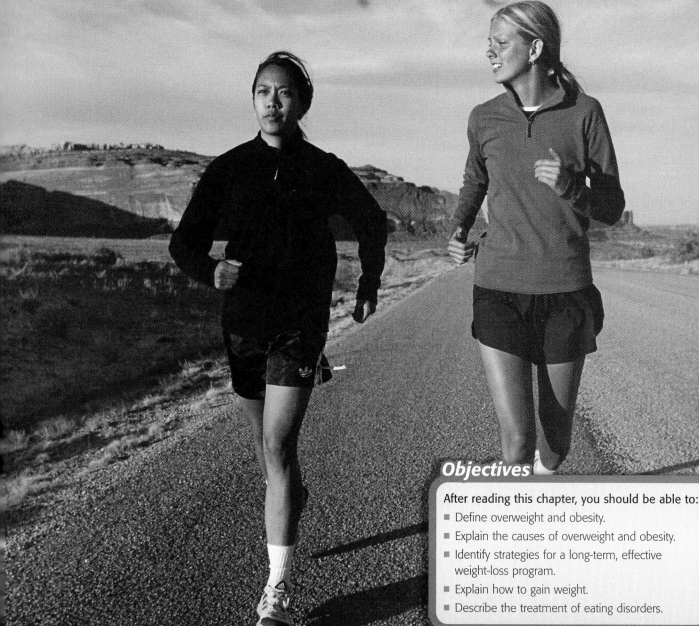

Objectives

After reading this chapter, you should be able to:

- Define overweight and obesity.
- Explain the causes of overweight and obesity.
- Identify strategies for a long-term, effective weight-loss program.
- Explain how to gain weight.
- Describe the treatment of eating disorders.

How Much Do You Need to Eat?

Do you want to lose weight, or keep it where it is? Don't know where to start?

Here's a quick way to find out how many calories you currently need.

What Do I Need to Begin?

Your basal metabolic rate (BMR) is the amount of energy your body needs to keep you breathing, to keep your heart beating, and to maintain your body temperature. Believe it or not, your BMR accounts for about 70% of the total daily calories you expend. The rest is used by digestion and your daily physical activity.

What Benefits Will I Receive?

Just knowing your energy needs now will help you get started on a weight-loss or weight-management program.

What Do I Do?

Determine your calories-per-day energy need using **Table 8.1**.

Table 8.1	BMR Chart

Step 1: Find the equation appropriate for you and calculate your BMR.

Age	Males	Females
18–30	6.95 × body weight (lbs) + 679	6.68 × body weight (lbs) + 496
30–60	5.27 × body weight (lbs) + 879	3.95 × body weight (lbs) + 829

Your BMR is _____ calories/day.

Step 2: Find your physical activity factor below.

Activity level	Description	Activity factor
Sedentary	Mostly resting with little or no activity	1.2
Light	Occasional unplanned activity (e.g., going for a walk)	1.4
Moderate	Daily planned activity, such as a brisk walk or bicycling	1.6
Heavy	Daily workout routine requiring several hours of continuous exercise	1.9
Exceptional	Daily, vigorous workouts for extended time period; training for competition	2.3

Step 3: Multiply your BMR calories by your activity factor to find your daily energy requirement:

_____	×	_____	=	_____
Your BMR		Your activity factor		Your calories/day energy need

What's the word. . .

calorie Unit of energy supplied by food; equals 1 kilocalorie (kcal), the amount of heat required to raise the temperature of 1 kilo of water 1°C.

basal metabolic rate (BMR) Energy consumed (measured in calories) by the body at rest to keep vital functions going.

8

Obesity

Over 60% of adults in the United States are either overweight or obese (NCHS 2004). The obesity epidemic covered on television and in newspapers did not occur overnight. Obesity and overweight are chronic conditions. Overall, there are a variety of factors that play a role in obesity (NCCDPHP 2001).

Individuals with a BMI of 25 to 29.9 are considered overweight, while individuals with a BMI of 30 or more are considered obese. NOTE: Overweight may or may not be due to increases in body fat. It may also be due to an increase in lean muscle. For example, professional athletes may be very lean and muscular, with very little body fat, yet they may weigh more than others of the same height. While they may qualify as "overweight" due to their large muscle mass, they are not necessarily "over fat," regardless of BMI (NCCDPHP 2004).

The concern regarding body fat include both the distribution of fat throughout the body and the size of the adipose tissue deposits. Body fat distribution can be estimated by skinfold measures, waist-to-hip circumference ratios, or techniques such as ultrasound, CT, or MRI scans (NCCDPHP 2004).

What Causes Weight Gain

Your weight changes depend on a simple rule:

When the number of calories consumed is not equal to the number of calories used, the following occurs:

Calories Consumed > Calories Used = **Weight Gain**

Calories Consumed < Calories Used = **Weight Loss**

Calories Consumed = Calories Used = **No Weight Gain**

See **Figure 8.1**.

(a) Energy is in balance.

(b) Energy intake is less than energy expenditure.

(c) Energy intake exceeds energy expenditure.

Figure 8.1

The balance between energy intake and expenditure controls weight management.

Health Risks of Too Much Body Fat

The main concern about overweight and obesity is one of health and not appearance (Figure 8.2). Too much storage fat is unhealthy.

Obese people are at a higher risk for diabetes, heart disease, stroke, high blood pressure, and premature death. They are also prone to gallbladder disease, arthritis, varicose veins, and shortness of breath (Table 8.2).

Premature Death

- The risk of premature death rises with increasing weight.
- Obese individuals are at a 50–100% increased risk of death from all causes.

Heart Disease

- High blood pressure is twice as common in obese adults.
- Obesity is associated with elevated triglycerides (blood fat) and decreased HDL (good) cholesterol.
- Heart disease (heart attack, congestive heart failure, sudden cardiac death, chest pain, and abnormal heart rhythm) is increased in those who are overweight or obese.

Diabetes

- More than 80% of people with type 2 diabetes are overweight or obese.
- A weight gain of 11 to 18 pounds increases a person's risk of developing type 2 diabetes to twice that of individuals who have not gained weight.

Cancer

- Overweight and obesity are associated with an increased risk for some types of cancer, including endometrial (cancer of the lining of the uterus), colon, gallbladder, prostate, kidney, and postmenopausal breast cancer.
- Women gaining more than 20 pounds from age 18 to midlife double their risk of post menopausal breast cancer.

Figure 8.2

Type 2 diabetes (noninsulin dependent)
Back pain
Heart disease (coronary and congestive)
Stroke
Asthma; shortness of breath
Cancer (endometrial, colon, prostate, kidney, gallbladder, and postmenopausal breast cancer)
Bladder control problems (stress incontinence—urine leakage caused by weak pelvic-floor muscles)
Hypertension (high blood pressure)
High blood cholesterol
Premature death
Complications of pregnancy
Gallbladder disease (gallstones)
Menstrual irregularities
Osteoarthritis (degeneration of cartilage and bone in joints)
Increased surgical risk
Sleep apnea (intermittent cessation of breathing while sleeping) and respiratory problems
Psychological disorders (e.g., depression, eating disorders, distorted body image, low self-esteem)

Health risks for overweight and obese people.

Table 8.2	Health Risks Associated with Obesity
Obesity is associated with an increased risk of:	

- Premature death	- High blood cholesterol
- Type 2 diabetes	- Complications of pregnancy
- Heart disease	- Menstrual irregularities
- Stroke	- Hirsuitism (presence of excess body and facial hair)
- Hypertension	- Stress incontinence (urine leakage caused by weak pelvic-floor muscles)
- Gallbladder disease	
- Osteoarthritis (degeneration of cartilage and bone in joints)	
- Sleep apnea	- Increased surgical risk
- Asthma	- Psychological disorders, such as depression
- Breathing problems	- Psychological difficultires due to social stigmatization
- Cancer (endometrial, colon, kidney, gallbladder, and postmenopausal breast cancer)	

Source: Surgeon General's Call to Action to Prevent and Decrease Overweight and Obesity, 2001.

Adapted from www.niddk.nih.gov/health/nutrit/pubs/statobes.htm.

8

Breathing Problems

- Sleep apnea (interrupted breathing while sleeping) is more common in obese persons.
- Obesity is associated with a higher prevalence of asthma.

Arthritis

For every two-pound increase in weight, the risk of developing arthritis is increased by 9% to 13%. But symptoms of arthritis can improve with weight loss.

Additional Health Consequences

- Overweight and obesity are associated with increased risks of gallbladder disease, incontinence, surgical complications, and depression.
- Obesity can affect the quality of life through limited mobility and decreased physical endurance, as well as through social, academic, and job discrimination.

Pregnancy and Childbirth

- Obesity during pregnancy is associated with increased risk of death in both the baby and the mother, and increases the risk of maternal high blood pressure by a factor of 10.
- Obese women are more likely during pregnancy to have gestational diabetes and problems with labor and delivery.
- Infants born to women obese during pregnancy are more likely to be high in birth weight and low in blood sugar (associated with brain damage and seizures).
- Obesity during pregnancy is associated with increased risk of birth defects, particularly neural tube defects such as spina bifida.
- Obesity in premenopausal women is associated with irregular menstrual cycles and infertility.

Children and Adolescents

- Risk factors for heart disease, such as high cholesterol and high blood pressure, occur with increased frequency in overweight children and adolescents compared to those with a healthy weight.
- Type 2 diabetes (noninsulin dependent), previously considered an adult disease, has increased dramatically in children and adolescents. Overweight and obesity are closely linked to type 2 diabetes.
- Overweight adolescents have a 70% chance of becoming overweight or obese adults. This increases to 80% if one or more parent is overweight or obese.
- Obese people are more likely to have accidents, because they can't move easily.
- Obese people are socially and occupationally stigmatized, and generally have lower self-esteem.

Factors Contributing to Obesity

Many factors influence what and when you eat and how many calories you burn.

Early Theories of Weight Gain

Fat Cell Theory

Fat cell theory says that obesity is related to too many fat cells and enlarged fat cells. People with an above-average number of fat cells may have been born with them or may have developed them at certain times because of overeating. Restricting calories only decreases the size of fat cells, not the number.

Set Point Theory

Set point theory states that obese individuals are "programmed" to carry a certain amount of weight. This programming originates from a weight regulatory mechanism in the brain's hypothalamus. Even if you lose weight, your body strives to get back to its set point. To lose weight, the set point must be changed.

Glandular Disorder Theory

Hypothyroidism is the cause of only 1–2% of all over-weight (Insel 2002).

Current Theories About Weight Gain

Many factors influence weight gain. Some may start very early in life.

Genetics

Some individuals are genetically predisposed to gain weight more easily than others, or to store fat around the abdomen and chest. Children of overweight or obese parents, particularly the biological mother, are likely to develop weight problems (NCCDPHP 2001).

Diseases and Drugs

Some illnesses may lead to obesity or weight gain. These may include Cushing's disease, and polycystic ovary syndrome. Drugs such as steroids and some

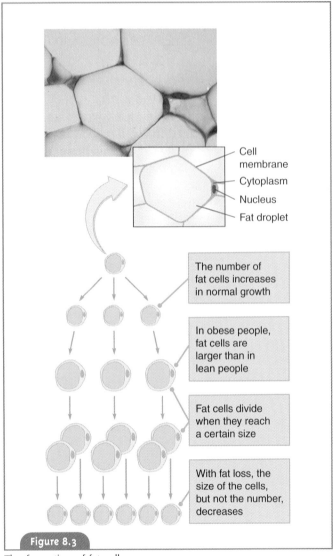

Cell membrane
Cytoplasm
Nucleus
Fat droplet

The number of fat cells increases in normal growth

In obese people, fat cells are larger than in lean people

Fat cells divide when they reach a certain size

With fat loss, the size of the cells, but not the number, decreases

Figure 8.3

The formation of fat cells.

antidepressants may also cause weight gain. A doctor is the best source to tell you whether illnesses or medications are contributing to weight gain or making weight loss difficult (NCCDPHP 2001).

Calorie Consumption

In the United States, a changing environment has broadened food options and eating habits. Grocery stores stock their shelves with a greater selection of products. Prepackaged foods, fast-food restaurants, and soft drinks are more accessible. While such foods are fast and convenient, they also tend to be high in fat, sugar, and calories. Choosing many foods from these categories can contribute to an excessive calorie intake. Some foods are marketed as healthy, low-fat, or fat-free, but may contain a lot of calories. It is important to read food labels for nutritional information and to eat in moderation (NCCDPHP 2001).

Portion size has also increased. People may be eating more during a meal or snack because of larger portion sizes (Figure 8.4). This results in increased calorie consumption. If the body does not burn off the extra calories consumed from larger portions, fast food, or soft drinks, weight gain can occur.

How do portions today compare to portions sizes 20 years ago? They are larger! The National Institutes of Health (NIH) developed a website (see website section at the end of this chapter) to inform people about the increasing portion sizes.

Some Rules: 72-ounce Steak

Rule #1 is to have fun. We really want you to win! The $50 dinner consists of a baked potato, salad, shrimp cocktail, roll, and a 72-ounce top sirloin steak. You must sit at the designated table in our dining room. You may not leave the table for any reason once the contest starts. No one may assist you in any way (such as cutting up your meal). You must complete the dinner in 1 hour (if you can't do the meal in an hour, you ain't going get it done in 2 hours anyway). You may not share your meal even if you don't complete the dinner (like take it back to your table to be shared by any folks you may have invited to cheer you on). If you get sick (its been known to happen) the contest is over, period. You can order the steak cooked any way you want. We will allow you a sample bite (small) prior to the start of the timer to make sure it is cooked to your satisfaction and the taste meets with your approval. Then we start the timer for one hour. You do not have to eat the fat or gristle (if you can find any), but we must judge this. Again, we want you to win but we do know our meats and will judge accordingly. The contest is just that, a contest. The steak is not offered on our menu as a meal. We do not allow the dinner to be ordered as a meal (unless you want to spend $200). It takes us a little more than a half an hour to cook the steak and it is available 365 days a year from 8:00am to 9:30pm. Enough with the rules! Refer to rule #1---HAVE FUN!

Figure 8.4

A well-known restaurant in Texas offers a contest for its patrons: eat a 72-ounce steak dinner in under an hour and it's free. These types of contests reinforce the fact that portion sizes for the American meal have increased to the point of being unhealthy. (*Source:* Photo and contest rules reproduced with permission by the Big Texan Steak Ranch. http://www.bigtexan.com/72oz.html.)

Calories Used

Our bodies need calories for functions such as breathing, digestion, and daily activities. Weight gain occurs when calories consumed exceed this need. For example, to lose one pound, decrease caloric intake by 3500 calories and maintain the same amount of activity, or increase physical activity to burn 3500 calories. Physical activity plays a key role in energy balance because it uses up calories consumed.

Despite all the benefits of being physically active, most Americans are sedentary. Technology has created many time- and labor-saving products. Some examples include cars, elevators, computers, dishwashers, and televisions. Cars are used to run short-distance errands instead of walking or riding a bicycle. As a result, these recent lifestyle changes have reduced the overall amount of energy expended in our daily lives (NCCD-PHP 2001). According to the Behavioral Risk Factor Surveillance System, in 2000, more than 26% of adults reported no leisure-time physical activity.

The belief that physical activity is limited to exercise or sports may keep people from being active. Another myth is that physical activity must be vigorous to achieve health benefits. Physical activity is any bodily movement that results in an expenditure of energy. Moderate-intensity activities such as household chores, gardening, and walking can also provide health benefits.

Socioeconomic, Age, and Gender Factors

- Age—Fatness increases during adulthood and declines in the elderly.
- Gender—Obesity is more prevalent in women than men.
- Culture—People in developed countries have more body fat than those in developing societies.
- Race/Ethnicity—Obesity is more prevalent in African American, Hispanic, Native American, and Pacific Islander people.
- Income—Obesity is more prevalent in lower-income women.
- Education—Less-educated women have a high incidence of obesity.
- Employment—Unemployed women have a higher incidence of obesity.
- Marriage—Married men have a higher incidence of obesity.
- Residence—Rural women have a higher incidence of obesity.
- Region—People living in the Southern states have a higher incidence of obesity (Insel 2002).

Psychological Factors

- Weight Cycling—This is a pattern of losing and regaining weight, over and over again (yo-yo dieting). Experts believe that despite potential risks, any successful effort to lose pounds, even if temporary, can have potential benefits.
- Restrained Eaters—This involves trying to reduce food intake by fasting or avoiding food as long as possible, usually by skipping meals or delaying eating. When emotionally stressed, the restrained eater overeats without realizing it.
- Binge Eaters—This involves compulsive overeating, sometimes for days. This behavior is common among people in weight-loss programs (Insel 2002).

Weight Management

Worldwide, the number of overweight or obese people has increased markedly in recent years. Over 60% of Americans are overweight or obese. Health problems from excess body fatness are a major concern. Obesity is a risk factor for many chronic diseases

8

including heart disease, cancer, hypertension, and diabetes. Surveys show that nearly half of all American women and a third of men are trying to slim down. **Weight management** is an annual multibillion dollar business (ADA 1997 and ACSM 2001).

Losing weight permanently is difficult. Studies show that 95% of all dieters regain their lost weight and go on to add more pounds. However, lessons can be learned from those who have been successful. Their successes prove that anyone can lose weight.

A *Consumer Reports* (2002) survey of more than 32,000 dieters on long-term weight-loss maintenance found that ordinary people can be successful without using expensive commercial diet programs, special foods, dietary supplements, or drugs. The successful people tended to adopt low-carbohydrate/high-protein diets, rather than low-fat diets, and exercised.

Most chose walking and a sizeable number added weight lifting. They also consumed lean protein with judicious amounts of healthful fats.

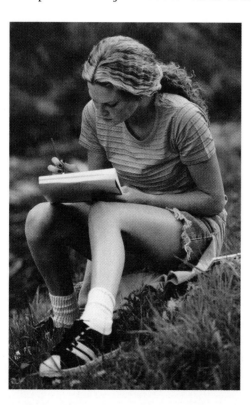

Where to Begin?

- Complete the body composition assessments found in Chapter 7. Take your photo in tight-fitting clothes. Attach a date to it. Keep this on hand as motivation.

- Set a realistic weight-loss goal. Most experts say it is reasonable to lose half a pound to two pounds a week. Some people lose more; some lose less. You have to burn 3500 calories more than you consume to lose one pound.

Studies show that dieters lose about 10% of their starting weight in the first 3 to 6 months (ACSM 2001 and NHLBI 1998). For those who weigh 200 pounds, that is about 20 pounds.

- Keep a food diary. Write down what you ate, how much you ate, when you ate, and whether you think you were overeating. Dieters who keep a daily food record usually lose more weight.

Exercise

- Increasing exercise while eating the same number of calories is not very effective for losing weight in the short term. To lose even a small amount of weight just by exercising, you have to exercise a lot. For example, to burn one pound of fat, you have to briskly walk or run 35 miles.

- The National Academies' Institute of Medicine's activity guideline (2002) says that, although health benefits are achieved from 30 minutes of activities, it takes an hour or more to prevent weight gain. Sedentary individuals can meet this goal by using moderate-intensity activity (e.g., walking at 4 miles per hour) for a total of 60 minutes on most days of the week, or engaging in a high-intensity activity (e.g., jogging, running) for 20 to 30 minutes 4 to 7 days per week.

- While vigorous exercise uses calories at a higher rate, any physical activity burns calories. For example, a 140-pound person can burn 175 calories in 30 minutes of moderate bicycling, and 322 calories in 30 minutes of moderate jogging. The same person can also burn 105 calories by vacuuming or raking leaves for the same amount of time.

- Some believe that dieting is better than exercise for weight reduction. It is easier to reduce caloric intake (refusing to eat a piece of cake with 250 calories) than it is to burn off the calories (jogging more than 2 miles at 100 calories per mile).

- Evidence clearly shows the need for activity in a weight-reduction program. Dieting can lead to weight loss, but the loss accompanies a greater loss of protein (lean tissue) and water. When lean tissue is lost, the body becomes less able to burn calories and more fat weight is eventually gained.

- Studies show that weight loss with exercise maximizes the removal of fat, minimizes the loss of protein, and helps maintain the metabolic rate. Dieting alone is seldom effective over the long term. Most weight-loss diets fail and the person has more weight and fat than before the dieting began.

Certain cautions should be taken by overweight and obese persons during exercising:

- For maximum benefit and minimum risk, choose low-to-moderate intensity activities.

- Ease into an exercise program. Increase the duration and frequency of exercise before increasing the intensity.

- Include strength training to build or maintain lean muscle.

The Inside Track

Use a Step Counter

For several years, researchers and public-health officials have encouraged people to walk at least 10,000 steps a day, which is roughly five miles. Children should be moving even more. But most Americans take an average of 5300 steps in a day.

Those who are overweight tend to walk 1500 to 2000 steps a day fewer than those who are not overweight. Moving 2000 steps a day, which is about one mile and should take about 15 to 20 minutes, burns 100 calories (depending on your height) (NHLBI 1998 and Hill et al. 2004).

Table 8.3	Guide for Losing Weight
Starting weight (in pounds)	Number of daily calories
<180	1500
180–215	1600
216–250	1800
250>	2000

Eat Fewer Calories

Your diet should be low in calories, but not too low (e.g., less than 800 kcal/day). Those lower than 800 kcal/day have been found to be no more effective than low-calorie diets in producing weight loss.

This chapter's Quick Start provides a means for determining the number of calories you need to maintain your current weight. To lose weight, try to eat 300 to 500 fewer calories than you need and to exercise 30 to 60 minutes on most days of the week.

Table 8.3 is a general guide to the number of calories you might want to consume if you are trying to lose a half-pound to two pounds a week.

Cut Back on Sugars (Carbs)

The body's use of carbohydrates seems to be the key to weight mangement. Eating foods that make your blood-sugar and insulin levels shoot up and then crash may contribute to weight gain. Such foods include white bread, white rice, other highly processed grain products, and potatoes. As an alternative, choose foods that have a gentler effect on blood sugar (called a low-glycemic-index; see Chapter 6 for more information). These include whole grains such as whole-grain breads and pasta, oats, as well as beans, nuts, fruits, and vegetables.

Eat Lean Protein

Eating lean protein includes reduced-fat dairy products, egg whites, fish, chicken, and lean cuts of beef and pork. Adding protein to the diet slows the absorption of food—blood-sugar will rise more slowly. You will not be as hungry.

Eating more protein and fewer carbohydrates has become a popular dieting approach. The long-term effects of eating this way on weight and overall health need further study. Such a diet might cause kidney damage in some people and rob bones of calcium. Avoid protein containing saturated and trans fats.

Eat Fruits and Vegetables

Fruits and vegetables are clearly an important part of a good diet. Almost everyone can benefit from eating more of them. They also provide fiber. Some experts recommend at least nine servings a day rather than the often recommended five servings. Choose a variety that includes dark-green, leafy vegetables; yellow, orange, and red fruits and vegetables; cooked tomatoes; and citrus fruits. Try to avoid fruit juices because they are high in calories.

Eat High-Fiber Grains and Legumes

This type of eating includes oatmeal, brown rice, whole-wheat bread, and lentils. You can trick your stomach into feeling full before you have eaten too many calories. Just drinking water does not give the stomach a full feeling; the water has to be part of the food. Examples of foods with the lowest energy density include: water-rich fruits and vegetables, whole grains, and lean meats.

Include Small Amounts of Healthful Fats

Examples of healthful fats are olive oil, avocadoes, nuts, olives, and fatty fish (e.g., salmon). Fat in a meal, or in snacks such as nuts, helps you feel full. Actually, eating certain healthful kinds of fats—mono- and polyunsaturated vegetable oils, nuts, and fish oil—seems to protect people against heart disease. Once again, avoid saturated and trans fats.

Other Strategies

Avoid overeating by using these tactics:

- Limit or avoid desserts—anything with simple sugars and/or refined carbs: all calories and not much nutrition.
- Eat slowly; eat at regular times; enjoy your food.
- Eat smaller portions; use small plates and bowls.
- Keep a food log—know how many calories you are eating.
- Eat a healthy snack before mealtime to curb your appetite.
- Stop eating before you feel full; you do not have to eat everything.
- Keep tempting food out of sight.

Weight Loss Options to Avoid

Using a Diet Book

Be wary of diet books, especially those recommending a single food, such as grapefruit or cabbage, or an imbalance of foods. The problem with following a special diet of the kind usually found in popular diet books is that it is difficult to stay with it. Once you backslide, you regain weight, and that can be really discouraging.

Better to permanently change the way you eat, with balance and good sense, taking your own weaknesses into account, but with moderation. That is the kind of diet you are most likely to stick with, be successful with, and be happy about.

Diet Supplements

Diet supplements are the new snake oil. They promise the easy way out, but cannot guarantee it. In fact, they are sold as supplements so they can steer clear of government regulation, and some are unsafe.

Can you live the rest of your life on a diet drink? Not likely. To get a quick weight loss (mainly muscle mass) you are substituting a diet supplement for the range of nutrients you need and can get from a healthy, balanced diet.

There is no good shortcut to healthy and sustainable weight loss.

Medical Help

If you are obese, and need serious help, a hospital- or clinic-based program may be your best approach. There you will be put on a medically supervised and closely monitored diet designed to get you back to a healthy weight.

Prescription Drugs

There are prescription drugs available that help people lose weight. Only two of them are approved by the FDA: one to suppress appetite, and the other to block fat absorption in the small intestine.

Other drugs, such as those that increase the metabolic rate, are not recommended—and even unsafe: Some weight-loss drugs have been found to cause potentially fatal heart problems. Even if safe, it is not a good idea to depend on drugs alone. Proper diet and exercise are still the real answer.

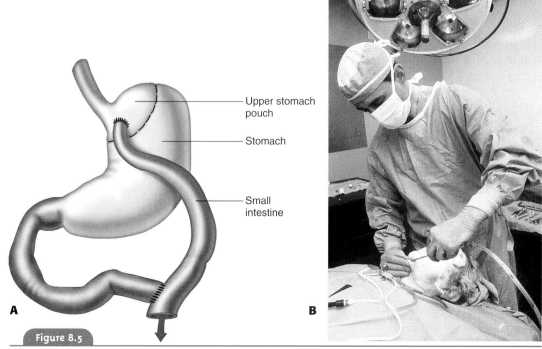

Figure 8.5

A. Gastric bypass surgery is a surgical procedure used to treat obesity. After surgery, the obese person experiences discomfort after overeating and is less likely to overeat. **B.** Liposuction has gained popularity in recent years.

Surgery

A growing number of people who find it impossible to change their eating and non-exercise habits have turned to surgery to change their bodies. The very obese who cannot control their appetites are often candidates. Surgical approaches to weight control should be considered only as a last resort for the obese.

A popular but potentially risky procedure is gastric bypass **Figure 8.5A**. The stomach is divided into two parts, using staples, and one is a small pouch for food. The patient feels full after eating only a small amount, and cannot eat more without getting sick.

A related surgical technique is resectioning the intestines so that only a small amount of food is digested.

A third method is liposuction, in which subcutaneous fat is suctioned away **Figure 8.5B**. This is intended for body reshaping, not weight loss.

Underweight

Underweight is not as common as overweight. When being underweight is inherited, and diet and other health behaviors are fine, the health risk is not a problem.

If the cause is not hereditary, and underweight is the result of undernutrition, deficits in protein and other nutrients as well as energy can cause disorders ranging from fatigue and problems with reproduction in women, to susceptibility to disease.

Causes of Underweight

- Hereditary and metabolic factors
- Prolonged psychological and emotional stress
- Addiction to alcohol and illicit drugs
- Inadequate or bizarre diets
- Eating disorders, compulsive dieting, and compulsive overexercising
- An underlying disease (e.g., cancer) (Insel 2002)

How to Gain Weight

Gaining weight can be difficult, but the basic concepts of energy balance apply. For example, to gain one pound, increase daily caloric intake by 3500 calories and maintain the same amount of activity.

- Eat small frequent meals.
- Eat snacks between meals.
- Eat high caloric foods and drinks.
- Eat extra servings of white bread, cereal, white rice, and pasta.
- Exercise to increase muscle mass.
- Use a balanced vitamin/mineral supplement to ensure deficiency does not contribute to poor appetite.

> **The Inside Track**
>
> **Who Should NOT Attempt Weight Loss?**
>
> - Most pregnant women
> - Most lactating (breast-feeding) women
> - Those with a serious, uncontrolled psychiatric illness (e.g., major depression)
> - Those who have any serious illnesses that would be complicated or worsened by caloric restriction
> - Those actively engaged in substance abuse
> - Those with a history of anorexia or bulimia (they should seek specialized care)

Eating Disorders

Eating disorders are a severe psychological response to body image issues. They occur mainly among high-achievement–oriented girls and young women (Figure 8.6).

They see themselves as overweight even though they are dangerously thin. Unusual eating habits develop: avoiding food and meals, and picking out a few foods and eating these in small quantities.

Anorexia Nervosa

Anorexia nervosa is an obsession for thinness manifested in self-imposed starvation. Those suffering from anorexia nervosa develop emaciated bodies. This condition can be fatal if left untreated. Also, about 25% of anorexics exercise compulsively to stay lean (Figure 8.7).

Related to anorexia is female athlete triad, an increasingly common condition among female athletes (Figure 8.8). The symptoms and results include amenorrhea and osteoporosis.

> **What's the word. . .**
>
> **eating disorder** A spectrum of abnormal eating patterns that eventually may endanger a person's health or increase the risk for other diseases. Generally, psychological factors play a key role.
>
> **anorexia nervosa** Extreme restriction of food intake.
>
> **female athlete triad** Combination of eating disorders, amenorrhea, and osteoporosis.
>
> **amenorrhea** Absence of normal menstruation.

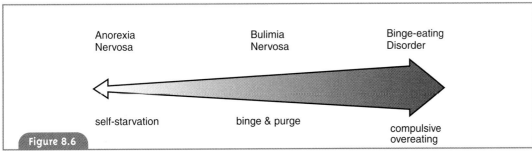

Figure 8.6

Eating disorder continuum.

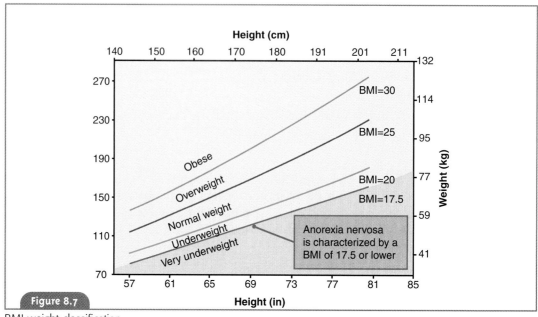

Figure 8.7

BMI weight classification.

Bulimia and Binge Eating

Bulimia and binge eating are often done by people who are depressed and impulsive, usually when they are angry, sad, bored, or worried **Figure 8.9**. In both of these conditions, people eat more food than is typically eaten.

Bulimics binge by periodically eating large amounts of food, then purge by forced vomiting or use of laxatives. Another method is bingeing one day and starving the next day.

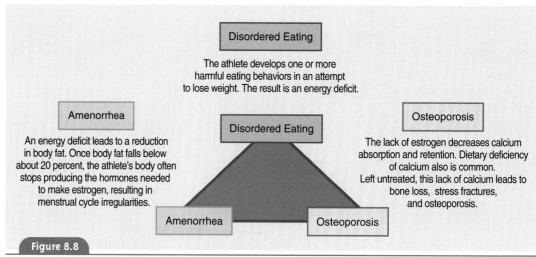

Figure 8.8

Stress fractures are a red flag for female athlete triad.

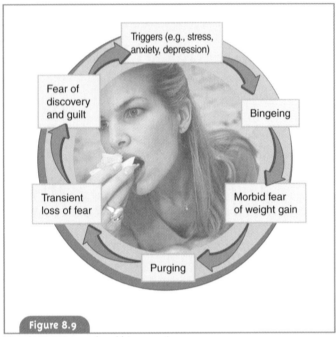

Figure 8.9
The destructive cycle of binge eating.

Treating Eating Disorders

Serious eating disorders, such as anorexia and bulimia, are very difficult to treat successfully. People with eating disorders deny them, and are secretive about them. If you are a friend or family member who wants to help, here is where to start:

- Tell the person you are concerned about their weight loss.
- Encourage the person to discuss with you any problems or anxieties.
- Make no judgments.
- Urge the person to see a professional—counselor, doctor, or psychologist.
- Talk to a counselor to see if intervention is possible—and about your own feelings, if you are very distressed yourself over the situation.

Professional treatment for eating disorders is a must. Usually a combination of overall supervision by a physician, medication such as an antidepressant, and psychotherapy are required.

Reflect ›››› **Reinforce** ›››› **Reinvigorate**

Knowledge Check

Answers in Appendix D

1. When you are trying to lose weight, which of the following is the most effective way to shed unwanted pounds?

   A. Cut out all of the empty calories in your diet (candy, white bread, soda) and be involved in moderate activity (walking for 30 minutes 4 days a week)

   B. Exercise 4 days a week very intensely (30-minute jog) while keeping the same diet

   C. Do more household chores, such as vacuuming, raking, and washing dishes, while maintaining the same diet

2. While reading about the different reasons for weight gain, you learned about three different theories on excessive weight gain. Which theory says that everyone has a set number of fat cells and that when you lose weight you are not decreasing the number of fat cells, but the actual size of the fat cell?

   A. Glandular disorder theory

   B. Set point theory

   C. Fat cell theory

3. Diet books seem to come and go. You see people on talk shows talking about one fad diet or another, and that is exactly what they are: fads. Which of the following reasons is why most of these fad diets do not work?

   A. These diets do not generate the results that they claim they can

   B. They often involve extreme changes to your lifestyle that are difficult (and possibly unsafe) to maintain

   C. They don't take into account your caloric intake

Modern Modifications

Keep a Food Diary

Track your eating habits for the next couple days. Record:

- What you eat
- How much you eat
- When you eat—Try to associate it with an event (i.e., 3pm break between classes)
- Why you eat—Was it lunch time? Were you just hungry? Were you stressed or bored?
- How did you feel after? Satisfied? Still hungry? Guilty?

Critical Thinking

Answers in Appendix D

Scenario One: Paul gained 12 pounds in his first year out of college. He has been working long hours at his new job and has no time for exercise. He has been eating one or more meals at various fast-food restaurants each day.

1. Which is the *least* likely explanation for Paul's weight gain?

    A. Inactivity
    B. Glandular disorder
    C. Consuming too many calories

2. Which choice seems the most logical for Paul to use in losing weight?

    A. Have liposuction
    B. Take prescription drugs
    C. Increase physical activity and consume fewer calories

Scenario Two: Jolene has always been preoccupied with her weight. As far back as she can remember, she was fat. As an adult, she has tried every diet she has seen described in popular magazines.

3. Which is the most useful suggestion for Jolene to follow in losing weight?

    A. Include more fat in her meals to feel full afterward.
    B. Eat three large meals a day.
    C. Consume no more than 1200 calories a day.

4. In exercising to lose weight, which would you suggest for Jolene?

    A. Increase physical activity and also the number of calories consumed.
    B. Increase exercise and eat the same.
    C. Decrease the amount of calories consumed and increase physical activity.

5. What should Jolene set as her weight-loss goal?

    A. One to two pounds per week
    B. 20% of her present weight in six months
    C. Rapid weight loss—amount and time doesn't matter

Going Above and Beyond

Websites

American Obesity Association
http://www.obesity.org

American Dietetic Association
http://www.eatright.org

Center for Science in the Public Interest
http://www.cspinet.org

Centers for Disease Control and Prevention, Obesity and Genetics
www.cdc.gov/genomics/info/perspectives/obesity.htm

Fast Food Facts: Interactive Food Finder
http://www.olen.com/food

Frontline on Fat
http://www.pbs.org/wgbh/pages/frontline/shows/fat

MedlinePlus on Obesity Weight Loss
http://www.nlm.nih.gov/medlineplus/obesity.html
http://www.nlm.nih.gov/medlineplus/weightlossdieting.html

National Association of Anorexia Nervosa and Associated Disorders (ANAD)
http://www.anad.org

National Eating Disorders Association
http://www.nationaleatingdisorders.org

National Institutes of Health
hin.nhlbi.nih.gov/portion/

Office of Dietary Supplements
http://dietary_supplements.info.nih.gov

Shape Up America!
http://shapeup.org

USDA Food and Nutrition Information Center
http://www.nal.usda.gov/fnic

Weight Control Information Network
http://www.pueblo.gsa.gov/cic_text/health/weightloss4life/wtloss.htm

Weightloss2000
http://www.weightloss2000.com

References and Suggested Readings

ACSM. Position stand: appropriate intervention strategies for weight loss and prevention of weight regain for adults. *Medicine and Science in Sports and Exercise* 33(12)(2001):2145–2156.

ADA. Weight management: position of the American Dietetics Association. *Journal of the American Dietetics Association* 97(1997):71–74.

Anderson R. E. Exercise, active lifestyle, and obesity: making an exercise prescription work. *Physician and Sports Medicine* 27(10)(1999):41–50.

Foreyt J. P. An etiological approach to obesity. *Hospital Practice,* August 15, 1997: 123–148.

Hill, J.O. et al. *The Step Diet Book.* New York: Workman Publishing Company, Inc. 2004.

Insel P., Turner R. E., and Ross D. *Discovering Nutrition.* Sudbury, MA: Jones and Bartlett Publishers, 2003:268–270.

_____. *Nutrition.* Sudbury, MA: Jones and Bartlett Publishers, 2002:302–318.

Klem M. L., et al. A descriptive study of individuals successful at long-term maintenance of substantial weight loss. *American Journal of Clinical Nutrition* 66(1997):239–249.

NCCDPHP. *Defining Overweight and Obesity.* Atlanta, GA: NCCDPHP, 2004. [October 19, 2004]. http://www.cdc.gov/nccdphp/dnpa/obesity/defining.htm.

NCCDPHP. *Factors Contributing to Obesity.* Atlanta, GA: NCCDPHP, 2001. [October 19, 2004]. http://www.cdc.gov/nccdphp/dnpa/obesity/contributing_factors.htm.

NCHS. *Prevalence of Overweight and Obesity Among Adults:* United States, 1999–2002. Hyattsville, MD: NCHS, 2004. [October 19, 2004]. http://www.cdc.gov/nchs/products/pubs/pubd/hestats/obese/obse99.htm.

NHLBI. Clinical guidelines on the identification, evaluation, and treatment of overweight and obesity in adults. NIH Publication No. 98-4083(1998). http://www.nhlbi.nih.gov/guidelines/obesity/practgde.htm.

Rubinstein S. and Caballero B. Is Miss America an undernourished role model? *Journal of the American Medical Association* 283(12)(2000):1569.

The Truth about Dieting. *Consumer Reports* 2002; 67:26–31.

Stevens J., et al. The effect of age on the association between body-mass index and mortality. *New England Journal of Medicine* 338(1998):1–7.

Wickelgren I. Obesity: how big a problem? *Science* 280(1998):1364–1376.

Willett W.C. *Eat, Drink, and Be Healthy.* New York: Fireside, 2001:36–55.

Willett W.C. Guidelines for healthy weight. *New England Journal of Medicine* 341(1999):427–434.

Willett W.C. Is dietary fat a major determinant of body fat? *American Journal of Clinical Nutrition* 76(suppl)(1998):556s–562s.

CHAPTER 9

Managing Stress

Objectives

After reading this chapter, you should be able to:

- Explain stress, distress, and eustress.
- Identify common symptoms of stress.
- Describe common sources of stress.
- Describe strategies useful in coping with stress.

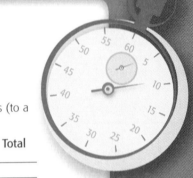

How Much Stress Have You Had Lately?

To estimate the amount of stress that you have endured recently, indicate the number of occasions (to a maximum of four) that you have experienced the following events in the past year.

Event	Number of Occasions	Points	Total
1. Death of a spouse	_____	87	_____
2. Marriage	_____	77	_____
3. Death of a close relative	_____	77	_____
4. Divorce	_____	76	_____
5. Marital separation	_____	74	_____
6. Pregnancy, or fathered a pregnancy	_____	64	_____
7. Death of a close friend	_____	68	_____
8. Personal injury or illness	_____	65	_____
9. Loss of your job	_____	62	_____
10. Breakup of a marital engagement or a steady relationship	_____	60	_____
11. Sexual difficulties	_____	58	_____
12. Marital reconciliation	_____	58	_____
13. Major change in self-concept	_____	57	_____
14. Major change in health or behavior of a family member	_____	56	_____
15. Engagement to be married	_____	54	_____
16. Major change in financial status	_____	53	_____
17. Major change in the use of drugs (other than alcohol)	_____	52	_____
18. Mortgage or loan of less than $10,000	_____	52	_____
19. Entered college	_____	50	_____
20. A new family member	_____	50	_____
21. A conflict or change in values	_____	50	_____
22. Change to a different line of work	_____	50	_____
23. A major change in the number of arguments with spouse	_____	50	_____
24. Change to a new school	_____	50	_____
25. A major change in amount of independence and responsibility	_____	49	_____
26. A major change in responsibilities at work	_____	47	_____
27. A major change in the use of alcohol	_____	46	_____
28. Revised personal habits	_____	45	_____
29. Being in trouble with school administration	_____	44	_____
30. A major change in social activities	_____	43	_____
31. Holding a job while attending school	_____	43	_____
32. Change of residence or living conditions	_____	42	_____
33. A major change in working hours or conditions	_____	42	_____
34. Trouble with in-laws	_____	42	_____
35. Your spouse beginning or stopping work outside the home	_____	41	_____
36. Change in dating habits	_____	41	_____
37. A change involving your major field of study	_____	41	_____
38. An outstanding personal achievement	_____	40	_____
39. Trouble with your boss	_____	38	_____
40. A major change in amount of participation in school activities	_____	38	_____
41. A major change in type and/or amount of recreation	_____	37	_____
42. A major change in religious activities	_____	36	_____
43. A major change in sleeping habits	_____	34	_____
44. A trip or vacation	_____	33	_____
45. A major change in eating habits	_____	30	_____
46. A major change in number of family get-togethers	_____	26	_____
47. Found guilty of minor violations of the law	_____	22	_____

Multiply the number of occasions times the point value for each event. Add the scores.

TOTAL POINTS _____

Your degree of stress is low if your score is lower than 347. If your score is higher than 1435, you are under a high degree of stress.

Source: Marx, M. B., Garrity, T. F., & Bowers, F. R. (1975). The influence of recent life experiences on the health of college students. Journal of Psychosomatic Research, 19:87-98. Used with permission.

What Is Stress?

Demands on your body that cause stress can be threats or challenges. Good **stress** (**eustress**) helps you perform better. Bad stress (**distress**) upsets you or makes you sick Figure 9.1 .

You feel distressed if you believe that:

- You have more problems than you can handle.
- You don't feel up to a task.

Exercising until you are exhausted is a physical **stressor**. Taking a tough exam is a mental stressor. Giving an in-class report is a social stressor. Being in a room filled with loud music is an environmental stressor. How you respond to the stressor is known as your **stress response**.

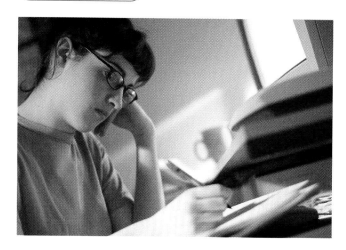

How Does Your Body Respond to Stress?

In response to stress, your body pours adrenaline, a stimulant hormone, into your bloodstream. The effects are:

- You sweat to cool the extra body heat and flush out body wastes.
- You hear and see better, to assess the situation and act quickly.
- Your heart speeds up, to get more blood to the muscles, brain, and heart.

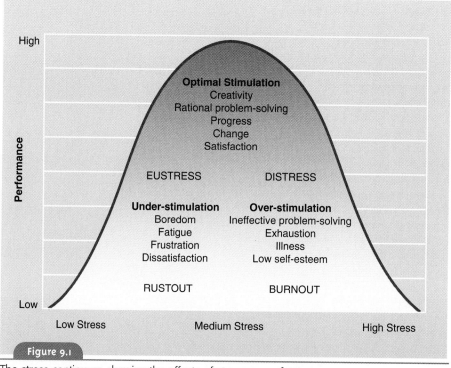

Optimal Stimulation
Creativity
Rational problem-solving
Progress
Change
Satisfaction

EUSTRESS   DISTRESS

Under-stimulation   **Over-stimulation**
Boredom   Ineffective problem-solving
Fatigue   Exhaustion
Frustration   Illness
Dissatisfaction   Low self-esteem

RUSTOUT   BURNOUT

High | Performance | Low

Low Stress   Medium Stress   High Stress

Figure 9.1

The stress continuum showing the effects of stress on performance.

- Blood flow increases to your brain, heart, and muscles, most important in dealing with danger.
- Your muscles tense to prepare for action.
- Less blood flows to your skin, digestive tract, kidneys and liver, least needed in times of crisis.
- You breathe faster, to take in more oxygen.
- Your liver dumps extra sugar, fats, and cholesterol into your bloodstream for quick energy.
- Platelets and blood-clotting factors rise to prevent hemorrhage in case of injury.
- Your body releases endorphins to mask pain.

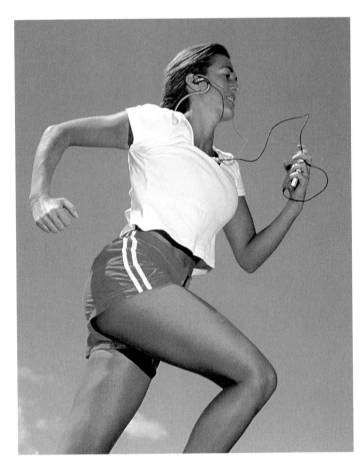

Endorphins are believed to be a source of "runner's high," an example of eustress.

How Does Your Nervous System React to Stress?

The sympathetic nervous subsystem of the autonomic nervous system triggers energy output to handle a crisis, including stress. It acts on almost all your organs, including your sweat glands, blood vessels, and muscles.

How Does Your Endocrine System React to Stress?

The endocrine system releases hormones to control body functions. In response to a stressor, it releases extra hormones from the adrenal gland, giving rise to the stress response.

What Is the Fight-or-Flight Response?

Adrenaline secreted into the bloodstream prepares the body for quick action during times of stress. The stress response is often called "fight-or-flight" because it either gets you ready to take action by staying and fighting or to run away from danger. Even in situations not requiring a physical response (e.g., being late for an in-class exam, having to stop at three red lights in a row, unable to find a parking space), the fight-or-flight response may be activated.

How Do You Return to Normal?

Once you have stopped stressing over something, the parasympathetic subsystem of your autonomic nervous system takes over and calms you down. It takes you back to homeostasis by bringing down your blood pressure, heart rate, and hormone levels, drying your sweaty palms, and slowing your breathing back to a normal pace.

What's the word. . .

endorphins Pain-inhibiting brain secretions.

sympathetic nervous system Subsystem of the autonomic system that triggers your body's response to stress—known as the fight-or-flight response.

autonomic nervous system Part of the nervous system that controls automatic body functions, such as blood pressure, heart rate, and breathing. Subdivided into sympathetic and parasympathetic.

endocrine system Consists of glands that produce hormones that control body functions.

hormone Chemical messenger released into the bloodstream that controls many body activities.

gland A group of cells that secretes hormones.

adrenaline A hormone that prepares the body to react during times of stress or in an emergency.

homeostasis Stability and consistency of a person's physiology.

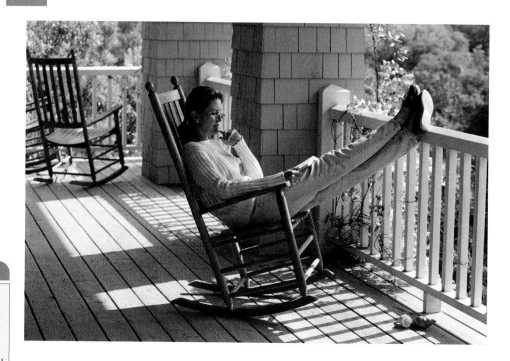

type A An individual exhibiting a sense of time urgency ("hurry sickness"), aggressiveness, and competitiveness, usually combined with hostility. Describes a great majority of Americans.

type B An individual displaying no sense of time urgency, no hostility, noncompetitiveness, patience, and a secure sense of self-esteem.

Personality Types and Stress

Certain kinds of behavior can aggravate the effects of stress. Extreme type-A people are at risk of coronary problems, unless they are able to channel their drive in constructive ways, and keep themselves in good physical shape.

Type-B people take things easy, do not respond to pressure or hurry, and do not set deadlines for themselves. They have a secure sense of self-esteem. However, an extreme type-B person may be avoiding life's challenges and as a result may not accomplish much.

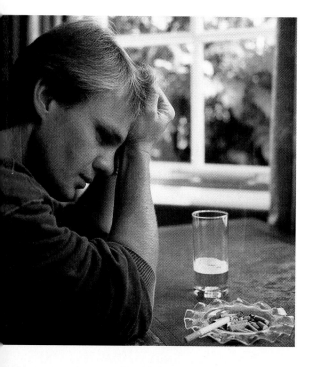

Ineffective Responses to Stress

Behavioral Responses

- Pacing and fidgeting, nail-biting, foot-tapping
- Overeating, smoking, drinking too much
- Crying, yelling, swearing, blaming other people and things
- Throwing things or hitting someone

Mental Responses

- Decreased concentration and memory
- Mind racing or going blank, confusion, indecisiveness
- Loss of sense of humor

Emotional Responses

- Anger and frustration, short temper, irritability, impatience
- Anxiety, nervousness, worry, fear
- Boredom, general fatigue, depression, low self-esteem

Stress and Disease

Of all illnesses, 50% to 80% relate to stress. The top-selling drugs in the United States are for stress-related disorders. According to the American Academy of Family Physicians, two thirds of all medical office visits are for stress-related illnesses **Figure 9.2**.

General Adaptation Syndrome

The general adaptation syndrome to stress (alarm, resistance, exhaustion) was first described by Dr. Hans Selye, a biologist **Figure 9.3**.

In the *alarm* stage, the first stage, the body prepares for quick action. The adrenal glands secrete adrenaline into the bloodstream, which prepares the body to deal physically with the stressor.

In the *resistance* stage, the second stage, the body attempts to regain internal balance. The body is no longer in the emergency state. Adrenaline is no longer secreted.

The first two stages are normal and healthful. However, some people are not able to manage stress. As a result, their bodies are in the alarm stage for long periods of time. The *exhaustion* stage, the third stage, represents the wearing on the body that increases

What's the word. . .

general adaptation syndrome A series of body changes that result from stress. The syndrome occurs in three stages: alarm, resistance, and exhaustion.

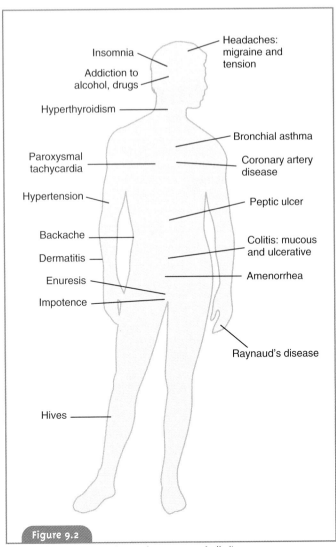

Figure 9.2
Stress relates to an estimated 50-80% of all diseases.

Figure 9.3

There are three stages of general adaptation syndrome. (a) In the alarm stage, the body's normal resistance to stress is lowered from the first interaction with the stressor. (b) In the stage of resistance, the body adapts to the continued presence of the stressor and resistance increases. (c) In the stage of exhaustion, the body loses its ability to resist the stressor any longer and becomes exhausted, the body's defenses weakened.

What's the word...

allostatic load The ongoing demand on the body from long-term exposure to stress hormones.

psychoneuroim-munology Study of nervous, endocrine, and immune systems interaction.

the risk of illness and premature death. Experts call the long-term wear of the stress response the **allostatic load**. When you are unable to cope with stress due to the allostatic load, you become more susceptible to illnesses.

Psychoneuroimmunology

Depending on your body and mind's ability to cope with stress, you can develop some serious health problems as a result of chronic stress, especially in your circulatory and immune systems:

- High blood pressure and arteriosclerosis leading to stroke or heart attack
- Increased susceptibility to colds, infections, rheumatoid arthritis, cancer, herpes, HIV

Other health problems from poor response to stress can include:

- Rapid or irregular heart rate, chest pains
- Muscle aches or stiffness (especially in neck, shoulders, and low back)
- Temporomandibular joint dysfunction (TMJ)
- Tension or migraine headaches
- Flushing or sweating, trembling, fatigue, cold extremities
- Nausea, abdominal cramps, irritable bowel syndrome, ulcers, and colitis
- Bronchial asthma, allergies, insomnia

Sources of Stress

There are many negative and positive sources of stress in your life. They can be especially stressful if they come in clusters.

- *Life changes:* Accumulating 300 or more life change units within six months or 500 life change units within one year shows a high degree of recent life stress **Table 9.1**.

Table 9.1	The Recent Life Changes Questionnaire

Life event	Life change units Women	Men	Life event	Life change units Women	Men
Death of son or daughter	135	103	Engagement to marry	47	42
Death of spouse	122	113	Moderate illness	47	39
Death of brother or sister	111	87	Loss or damage of personal property	47	35
Death of parent	105	90	Sexual difficulties	44	44
Divorce	102	85	Getting demoted at work	44	39
Death of family member	96	78	Major change in living conditions	44	37
Fired from work	85	69	Increase in income	43	30
Separation from spouse due to marital problems	79	70	Relationship problems	42	34
			Trouble with in-laws	41	33
Major injury or illness	79	64	Beginning or ending school or college	40	35
Being held in jail	78	71	Making a major purchase	40	33
Pregnancy	74	55	New, close personal relationship	39	34
Miscarriage or abortion	74	51	Outstanding personal achievement	38	33
Death of a close friend	73	64	Troubles with co-workers at work	37	32
Laid off from work	73	59	Change in school or college	37	31
Birth of a child	71	56	Change in your work hours or conditions	36	32
Adopting a child	71	54	Troubles with workers whom you supervise	35	34
Major business adjustment	67	47	Getting a transfer at work	33	31
Decrease in income	66	49	Getting a promotion at work	33	29
Parents' divorce	63	52	Change in religious beliefs	31	27
A relative moving in with you	62	53	Christmas	30	25
Foreclosure on a mortgage or a loan	62	51	Having more responsibilities at work	29	29
Investment and/or credit difficulties	62	46	Troubles with your boss at work	29	29
Marital reconciliation	61	48	Major change in usual type or amount of recreation	29	28
Major change in health or behavior of family member	58	50	General work troubles	29	27
Change in arguments with spouse	55	41	Change in social activities	29	24
Retirement	54	48	Major change in eating habits	29	23
Major decision regarding your immediate future	54	46	Major change in sleeping habits	28	23
			Change in family get-togethers	28	20
Separation from spouse due to work	53	54	Change in personal habits	27	24
An accident	53	38	Major dental work	27	23
Parental remarriage	52	45	Change of residence in same town or city	27	21
Change residence to a different town, city, or state	52	39	Change in political beliefs	26	21
			Vacation	26	20
Change to a new type of work	51	50	Having fewer responsibilities at work	22	21
"Falling out" of a close personal relationship	50	41	Making a moderate purchase	22	18
Marriage	50	50	Change in church activities	21	20
Spouse changes work	50	38	Minor violation of the law	20	19
Child leaving home	48	38	Correspondence course to help you in your work	19	16
Birth of grandchild	48	34			

Source: Adapted from Miller, M. A., and Rahe, R. H. (1997). Life changes scaling for the 1990s. *Journal of Psychosomatic Research,* 43, 279–292, with permission from Elsevier Science.

- *Daily hassles:* Commuting, misplacing keys, mechanical breakdowns, money worries, arguments, lousy weather, waiting in long or slow lines, noise, bright lights, heat, violence, confined spaces

- *College-life stress:* Adjusting to a new locale, making new friends, keeping up with tougher academic work, taking exams, meeting deadlines, too much caffeine, not enough sleep, overloaded schedule, worry about earning money to live on or taking on loans to pay expenses

- *Job stress:* Rushed by tight schedules and deadlines; too much overtime taking away from personal life; concerns about job performance, job security, or money earned; interactions with co-workers, bosses, or customers; no input on how work is done; dealing with bureaucratic rules and regulations **Figure 9.4**

- *Social stress:* Changes in relationships with family and old friends, aggressive behavior from others, negative community pressures from ethnic or lifestyle prejudice and discrimination, difficulties in using English as a second language

- *Negative thought patterns:* Pessimistic thinking, self-criticism, overanalyzing situations and relationships

- *Personality difficulties:* Unrealistic expectations, taking things too personally, exaggerating, all-or-nothing or rigid thinking

Figure 9.4

An extreme example of job-related stress is working on the New York Stock Exchange. So many people have heart attacks there every year that the exchange has installed a defibrillator near the phone banks.

Key Strategies for Coping with Stress Effectively

Effective coping strategies are anything that helps change or reduce the stress or the perception of stress.

Time Management

- Rank tasks in order of importance. (See Lab 9-1, Activity 1 on Time Ranking.)
- Schedule tasks with a time period for each. Break your day into quarter-hour or half-hour segments. (See Lab 9-1, Activity 2 on Scheduling.)
- List your deadlines on a calendar or daily planner so that you can allow time to meet them.
- Delegate. Ask for help. Involve others in doing your low-priority tasks.
- Say "no" if demands seem unreasonable or you do not have time for them.
- Have a place for everything and put everything in its place.
- Schedule personal time each day for exercise, a hobby, meditation, or some other activity that improves your quality of life.
- Watch less television (limit yourself to 1 hour each night).

The Inside Track

Roadblocks to Effective Time Management

- *Time urgency:* Rushing to meet deadlines
- *Time juggling:* Trying to do more than one thing at a time
- *Procrastination:* Avoiding or putting off what should be done, from apathy or fear of failure
- *Perfectionism:* Obsessed with doing everything perfectly; getting caught up in details and not seeing the whole picture
- *Workaholism:* Spending too much time at work
- *Can't say "no":* Taking on responsibilities you don't have time for or can't handle in order to get approval or acceptance
- *Polyphasic thinking:* Being preoccupied with many thoughts at one time

Healthy Diet

- Eat a well-balanced diet of milk, whole grains, fruits, vegetables, fish, and poultry; eat slowly; eat less junk food.
- Take in less caffeine (e.g., coffee, tea, colas, too much chocolate). Caffeine generates a stress reaction in the body.
- Avoid "stress-reducing" supplements, such as those containing vitamins and amino acid compounds. They do not help reduce the effects of stress.

Exercise

Exercise is a good way to dissipate stress. Get regular exercise (at least 30 minutes, three times per week). Take a brisk walk, a run, or a bike ride.

Cardiovascular exercise flushes stress hormones out of the body. Otherwise, they pool in the body and cause havoc (e.g., cortisol destroys white blood cells). Regular cardiovascular exercise may contribute to an overall sense of relaxation.

Exercise may also combat emotional problems, such as depression, by increasing the level of endorphins, chemicals in the brain that seem to enhance a sense of well-being and relieve anxiety.

Sleep

Sleep reduces stress. Tired people do not cope well with stressful situations. If you get enough sleep, you feel better and are more resilient and adaptable.

Successful sleep is:

- waking naturally
- waking refreshed
- having plenty of daytime energy

The "power nap" or catnap is short (5 to 20 minutes) and can be rejuvenating. Many people don't get enough sleep, some by choice. But bad things happen when you are sleep deprived:

- You doze off in class.
- You can't focus on an exam.
- You risk serious injury by dozing off while driving or working.

Lack of sleep also adversely affects your health:

- You are at a greater risk of infection.
- You become moody.
- You have problems with memory.

When are you getting enough sleep? When you wake up naturally without an alarm clock, and feel alert during the day.

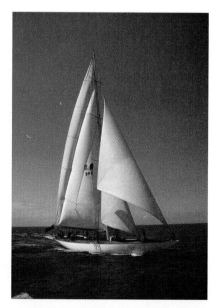

Social Support

Keep your connections to family and friends strong. When you are feeling stressed, talk to a family member, friend, counselor, school advisor, or teacher. You'll be surprised how much better you feel after talking to someone.

Healthy Thought Patterns

Attitude is crucial to stress management. In sailing terms, *attitude* is how sails are set to take advantage of prevailing winds. Thus, what we believe determines how we react to stress.

Positive thinking can help you manage stress. If you say to yourself, "I will ace that exam," you are more likely to do well and feel less stressed.

Communication: Managing Anger

Anger creates physical symptoms similar to stress: faster heartbeat and breathing, muscle tension, flushed face, and trembling. Out-of-control anger is bad for you. It hurts you and your relationships with others.

If you are angry:

- Reframe the situation. Maybe the cause isn't directed at you.
- Distract yourself. Count to ten. Imagine yourself in a peaceful place.
- Analyze the conflict. Listen to the other person's point of view. Negotiate a constructive solution.

If the other person is angry at you:

- Respond calmly.
- Ask why the person is angry.
- Focus on resolving the cause of the anger.
- If all else fails, disengage and try again later.

Additional Ways to Manage Stress

Music

Listening to and creating music has a soothing effect. For most people, music is a popular way to relax. To be fully effective as a relaxation technique, music should be instrumental, without lyrics.

Time-Outs

Take time-outs to get away from the things that are bothering you. This will decrease your stress levels.

Time-outs include power naps, meditation, daydreaming, a social conversation, a short walk, a refreshment break, or listening to music.

You have cycles throughout the day, peaks of energy and concentration interspersed with low energy and inefficiency. Watch for periods of low energy and take breaks when they occur.

A mid-morning break, lunch, a mid-afternoon break, and the evening meal divide a day into roughly 2-hour segments.

9

The relaxation response

Increased slow-brain-wave activity

Lowered oxygen consumption

Lowered blood pressure level

Increased skin resistance to electricity

Increased digestion

Figure 9.5

The relaxation response.

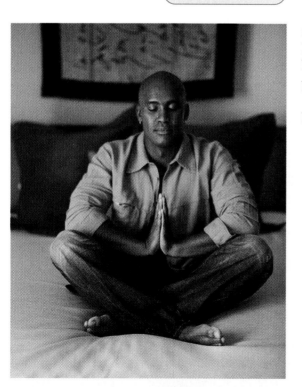

Relaxation Exercises

An effective relaxation technique is anything that helps reduce sensory overload by redirecting positive sensations through the five senses.

The Relaxation Response

The **relaxation response** is your ability to put your body into a state of deep relaxation (Benson 2000). All parts of the stress reaction are reversed: your pulse slows, your blood pressure falls, your breathing slows, and your muscles relax **Figure 9.5**.

The stress reaction is automatic. The relaxation response needs to be done deliberately. There are many ways of doing this:

- Sit quietly.
- Breathe from your diaphragm.
- Pet a dog or cat.
- Lie down on something comfortable, like a hammock.

Progressive Muscular Relaxation

Muscle tension is the most common symptom of stress. All ill people suffer from muscle tension. If you can reduce muscular tension, you become less susceptible to disease.

To combat stress, Edmund Jacobson developed a relaxation technique called **progressive muscular relaxation** (see Lab 9-2, Activity 1).

Meditation

Relaxation achieved through mediation is actually more physiologically restful than sleep. As little as 20 minutes once or twice per day provides significant benefit.

Basic steps (see Lab 9-2, Activity 2 on The Relaxation Response):

1. Find a quiet environment.
2. Take a comfortable position, usually sitting. Consciously relax the body's muscles.
3. Select a mental device (also known as a mantra). Try using the word *one*.
4. Close your eyes and inhale, then exhale. At the end of each exhalation say the mantra word (e.g., *one*) silently to yourself. Do this for 10 to 20 minutes.

Mental Imagery

Imagination can produce feelings of relaxation. For example, visualize yourself feeling warm, calm, and relaxed. Picture a tranquil setting that appeals to you and create a mental picture of the details (**Figure 9.6**).

- Mental imagery is generating images that have a calming, healing effect.
- Visualization is mental imagery consciously directed by yourself.
- In guided mental imagery, images are suggested by another person, either live or on tape.

Mental imagery can be used in a stressful situation (e.g., before making a public speech, at the start of an exam, waiting in line, sitting in a dentist's chair, during a meeting).

The technique can also be used to change your habits or better your perform-ance in various activities. Visualize, or imagine, yourself doing something differ-ently or performing successfully.

Yoga

Yoga, used since ancient times, can invigorate the body and calm the mind. Various postures, known as **asanas**, are performed in a specific sequence while breathing in a controlled manner. Yoga should be practiced for 15 to 45 minutes in a quiet place.

Figure 9.6

Visualize tranquil mental images to relax you when you are stressed.

Massage

Research indicates that human touch is vital for well-being. For example, infants require human touch to thrive. People of all ages need it as well.

All forms of massage tend to be both relaxing and invigorating. Massage requires the assistance of someone else to achieve full benefit.

Hydrotherapy (e.g., baths, hot tubs, jacuzzis, saunas) is another form of muscle massage.

What's the word. . .

asanas Various pos-tures used in doing yoga exercises.

9

Pets

Animals can offer more than just friendship, they can decrease stress levels as well. You will often find that hospitals and dentists have fishtanks—yes, even fish are capable of lowering our stress levels. The benefits of pet ownership have been studied a great deal; there have been numerous findings that pets lower their owners' blood pressure.

Sense of Humor

Humor may be the ultimate stress reliever. Studies show that humor promotes mental, emotional, physical, and spiritual well-being.

The author Norman Cousins, suffering from a connective tissue disease, credits his recovery to deliberate effort to apply humor to his situation.

When you try to find the humorous side of life, you can inoculate yourself against the hazards of stressful perceptions.

The average American laughs 15 times per day. Under stress, laughter drops to zero.

Think of some ways in which you can experience humor to lift your spirits (e.g., listening to a humorous radio program, sharing funny stories, reading cartoons).

Reflect >>>> Reinforce >>>> Reinvigorate
Knowledge Check
Answers in Appendix D

1. Good stress is called:
   A. Eustress
   B. Distress
   C. Stressful
   D. No stress
2. Which categories are manifest signs of stress?
   A. Physical (e.g., aches, stomach problems)
   B. Emotional (e.g., anxiety, boredom)
   C. Mental (e.g., indecisiveness, confusion)
   D. Behavioral (e.g., drinking, yelling, swearing)
   E. All of the above

Hobbies

Hobbies promote clear thinking. Take your mind off a problem and divert your attention to something else. When you return to the problem you will be better able to deal with it. Many people find that time spent pursuing hobbies helps generate solutions to life problems.

Hobbies provide pleasure and involve creativity. A hobby can boost self-esteem, which transfers to other areas of life.

Prayer

Prayer is one of the oldest and most commonly used methods of coping with life problems. If you are religious, prayer can promote mental and physical health.

A prayer commonly associated with stress seeks divine guidance or divine intervention. Such prayers are used when you need help yourself or when you pray for help to be given to others.

3. What are the three stages of the general adaptation syndrome:
   A. Flight, fright, sleep
   B. Confusion, hallucination, procrastination
   C. Alarm, resistance, exhaustion
   D. Anger, criticism, guilt

Modern Modifications

- Take 5 minutes each morning to visualize yourself being successful.
- Go for a brisk walk when you feel yourself becoming stressed during the day.
- Compile a CD with soothing music to listen to when you need to relax.
- Take a yoga class or rent a how-to video.
- Keep track of how many times you laugh in a day—if you are not laughing 15 times by the time you go to bed, try finding more humor in your life!

Critical Thinking

Answers in Appendix D

Scenario One: Dave was planning to go on a rafting trip next month, but has just been told that his trip is cancelled. A travel agent recommended by a friend had arranged the trip.

1. An appropriate way for Dave to reduce his stress would be to:
   A. Plan another vacation for the same time period
   B. Spend his vacation at home and read a book about river rafting
   C. Complain to his friend about his recommendation
   D. None of the above

Scenario Two: Maria has four final exams and only 2 days left to study for them.

2. An appropriate way for Maria to reduce her stress would be to:
   A. Take her mind off her own tests by helping a friend study
   B. Pick the hardest course and spend most of her time studying for that exam
   C. Set up a schedule so that she has some time to study for each test
   D. None of the above

Scenario Three: Greg lives across from an all-night service station and is disturbed by the traffic noise.

3. An appropriate way for Greg to reduce his stress would be to:
   A. Turn up his music to block out the noise
   B. Take a sleeping pill to help get to sleep
   C. Stay up later so that he can fall asleep more easily
   D. None of the above

Scenario Four: Joyce must speak to a large group of people. She is well prepared to give the speech. However, she keeps remembering another time when she gave a speech and forgot what she was supposed to say.

4. An appropriate way for Joyce to reduce her stress would be to:
   A. Set aside some time to sit quietly before the speech
   B. Look directly at the audience while she gives her speech
   C. Keep her hands busy while she gives the speech
   D. None of the above

Going Above and Beyond

Websites

American Institute of Stress
http://www.stress.org

American Psychological Association
http://www.apa.org http://helping.apa.org

The Humor Project
http://www.humorproject.com

National Institute for Occupational Safety and Health (NIOSH)
http://www.cdc.gov/niosh/stresshp.html

National Institute of Mental Health
http://www.nimh.nih.gov

National Sleep Foundation
http://www.sleepfoundation.org

References and Suggested Readings

Benson H. *The Relaxation Response.* New York: Avon/Wholecare, 2000.

Boscarino J. S. Diseases among men 20 years after exposure to severe stress: Implications for clinical research and medical care. *Psychosomatic Medicine 59*(1997):605–614.

Clements K. and Turpin G. Life event exposure, physiological reactivity, and psychological strain. *Journal of Behavioral Medicine 23*(1)(2000):73–94.

Friedman M. and Ulmer D. *Treating Type A Behavior and Your Heart.* New York: Knopf, 1984.

Laitinen J. E., et al. Stress-related eating and drinking behavior and body-mass index and predictors of this behavior. *Preventive Medicine 34*(1)(2002):29–39.

McKinney C. H., et al. Effects of guided imagery and music (GIM) therapy on mood and cortisol in healthy adults. *Health Psychology 16*(4)(1997):390–400.

Miller M. A. and Rahe R. H. Life changes scaling for the 1990s. *Journal of Psychosomatic Research 43*(1997):279–292.

Pashkow F. J. Is stress linked to heart disease? The evidence grows stronger. *Cleveland Clinic Journal of Medicine 66*(2)(1999):75–77.

Scheufele P. M. Effects of progressive relaxation and classical music on measurements of attention, relaxation, and stress responses. *Journal of Behavioral Medicine 23*(2)(2000):207–228.

Seaward B. L. *Managing Stress: Principles and Strategies for Health and Wellness,* 4th ed. Sudbury, MA: Jones & Bartlett Publishers, 2004.

Selye H. *The Stress of Life,* rev. ed. New York: McGraw-Hill, 1978.

Steptoe A. M. and Joekes K. Task demands and the pressures of everyday life: Associations between cardiovascular reactivity and work blood pressure and heart rate. *Healthy Psychology 19*(1)(2000):46–54.

Stephens T. Physical activity and mental health in the United States and Canada: Evidence from four population surveys. *Preventive Medicine 17*(1988):35–47.

Williams R. and Williams V. *Anger Kills.* New York: HarperCollins, 1993.

Responsible Decision Making

Objectives

After reading this chapter, you should be able to:

- Describe a lifetime fitness program.
- Evaluate a health/fitness club for reliability.
- Recognize myths and false claims about exercise nostrums.
- Assess exercise equipment before purchasing.
- List precautions to take when using hydrotherapy equipment/facilities.
- Identify exercise misinformation and quackery.

Being an Informed Consumer

The next time you watch a TV commercial or see a flyer for a quick weight loss program, take a moment to consider it. What is being said to you? Who is saying it? In today's day and age we find that in order to be healthy consumers we need to be educated consumers. The next time you see one of these ads, take a minute to answer the following questions:

- What claim is being made on behalf of this product?
- Who is making this claim? Is it an outside source or the company that makes the product?
- Is everything a testimony about how miraculous the product is?
- Does the ad list any studies that have been done to demonstrate the product's effectiveness?
- If yes, is this a credible source?
- Does it seem like a miracle cure or solution?
- How does it make you feel that products that may be noneffective or, worse, dangerous, are allowed to be marketed without any sound research?

This ad is merely a collection of value claims that are not supported by scientific research. The ad further attempts to encourage the reader to purchase the product by suggesting that it is better (and less expensive) than conventional therapies. It claims to relieve a wide range of health conditions. The red-flag phrases and testimonials rather than scientific evidence, the lack of details concerning the medical experts' credentials, and the lack of caution about the hazards of using the product all suggest the ad is an unreliable source of health-related information.

For centuries, doctors in the Orient have known about the wonders of herbal medicines—nature's botanical cures for human ailments.

PANACEA

All Natural

Finally, American scientists are recognizing the healthful benefits of these herbs.

SwayCon Pharmaceuticals has developed a capsule that contains everything you need to reduce suffering, enhance health, and regain youthful vigor.

A team of medical experts from three major medical schools in the United States have clinical proof that the ingredients of Panacea are effective! Panacea contains a chemical-free mixture of natural enzymes and exotic herbs that

- relieve up to 80% more arthritis pain than aspirin;
- lower blood pressure by up to 20%;
- lower cholesterol by up to 45%;
- reduce lung cancer risk by as much as 50%, even in smokers;
- and reduce the risk of heart attack by 75%.*

Other remarkable findings

Taking Panacea for a few months can improve intelligence. R.P., a college student at a large East Coast university reports, "At the beginning of the fall semester, I started taking three capsules of Panacea a day. My G.P.A. went from a 1.8 to a 3.4! Panacea has helped me get all A's!"

Reports are coming into our offices that Panacea acts as a sexual stimulant, increasing potency. S.D., a computer programmer in St. Louis, writes, "Thanks for saving my marriage. Before taking Panacea, my husband complained about my lack of interest in sex. One of my friends told me that Panacea can help. Just a few days after taking the capsules, our marriage turned into a perpetual honeymoon."

Panacea is only available in fine health food stores. Order a three-month supply now, while supplies last

* These statements have not been evaluated by the FDA.

"Clinical proof" is a red flag. The medical experts, the medical schools, or journals where their research has been published are not identified. Objective testing could show the product is neither safe nor effective. The ad should cite the specific effects of the product, including negative ones.

"Chemical-free" is a red flag; herbs, other plants, all matter is chemical. Furthermore, scientific studies should be cited to provide evidence for these value claims. These statements are not verifiable facts.

A testimonial from an individual is not scientific evidence. This student's G.P.A. my have risen for a variety of reasons. Studies conducted to show that a treatment is useful in particular ways should contain at least 30 subjects.

No scientific evidence is cited that a daily Panacea pill prevents serious illness. Additionally, this statement attacks conventional medical practitioners by implying that they are interested only in making money, which suggests that physicians can't be trusted.

Source: Alters, S. and Schiff, W. *Essential Concepts for Healthy Living,* 3rd edition. Sudbury, MA: Jones and Bartlett Publishers, 2003, p. 13.

Childhood to Old Age

What's the word. . .

endurance Ability to work out for a period of time without fatigue.

mall-walking Walking a circuit around the lobby floors of an enclosed shopping mall in the morning, often before the stores open.

t'ai chi Thirteenth-century Chinese exercise routine involving graceful dance-like movements.

If you expect to become a parent, bear this in mind: A physically active life begins in childhood. You will do your children no favors if you allow them to watch television or play computer games most of the time. Encourage children to balance those activities with sports, games, or other physical activity that they enjoy. Also, remember that as a parent you are a model for your child. Take time to do activities with your children to encourage them to spend time exercising.

Keep on exercising as you age. You'll have a healthier heart and fitter body. Exercise can reduce blood pressure, make your joints more flexible, and increase muscle strength and **endurance**. Not only your body benefits: You will improve your mood and your cognitive functions as well.

Keeping your balance as you age is a major issue. Falls that a young person bounces back from can incapacitate or be fatal for older people. Falls in old age are usually the result of poor balance, and keeping fit improves balance.

Even if you did not start early, you can start late. Light to moderate exercise will improve your health at any age: For example, **mall-walking**, dancing, **t'ai chi**, or fitness classes designed for older people.

College Students

Now is the time to make exercise a permanent part of your life. Most colleges try to make it convenient for you. Did you know the following?

- Your college or university probably offers a variety of fitness and sports courses and intramural athletic programs.
- College gyms and athletic fields are usually open at certain times for recreational student use and have some of the best trainers and equipment.

After College

It may take a bit more initiative, especially if your job is desk-bound, but you will be healthier if you create a personal program of physical activity and exercise after college.

Do activities you like; you are more likely to stick with them throughout your life.

There are some simple ways to make a difference in your daily physical activity:

- Walk to work, at least part of the way.
- Use the stairs, not the elevator.
- Walk during lunchtime.
- Ride a bicycle.

To be more serious about it, you can exercise at home, join a fitness club, or use the exercise facilities in your office building.

If you like to exercise at home, you can buy barbells and hand weights for resistance training, and for aerobic exercise, use a rowing machine, stationary bike, treadmill, stair climber, or cross-country ski machine. A great way to decide whether these are the best pieces of equipment to purchase for home use is to try them out at a fitness club before buying them.

If you like the social aspects of belonging to a fitness club or find it more motivating, by all means join one, but look before you leap.

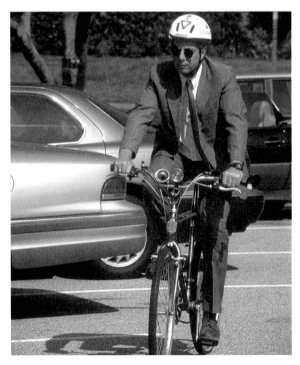

> **What's the word. . .**
> **resistance training**
> Building muscle by working against the resistance of weights.

How to Choose a Fitness Facility

Gyms offer a great number of resources and allow you access to expensive equipment and a variety of fitness classes. But be wary of a high-pressure sales pitch. Once you walk into a gym with one of their promotional fliers, the sales staff will do everything in their power to get you to join that day. Take some steps to find out if this is the best gym for you and then take some time to assess whether you can afford the membership.

- Find out how much it costs: Can you afford it? Never join a gym the first time you go. Ask to try out the club for a period of time before signing up. Then you can assess whether you will make the effort to go before making the financial investment.
- Check equipment quality and general cleanliness. Check out the changing rooms and showers.
- Interview the club's trainers. Ask for their credentials and names of clients you can call.

Tipping Point

Selecting a Fitness Professional Who Is Right for You

- Is the fitness professional's workspace convenient to your workplace or home, or is training available in your home?
- Are new clients provided with a pre-exercise screening for health-risk factors and is a fitness program designed specifically for their needs?
- Does the fitness professional offer the expertise, programs, and services you need to achieve your fitness goals?

- Ask them to describe a plan they might recommend for you.
- Ask how long the club has been in business.
- Check references. Talk to current clients, the Better Business Bureau, and the consumer protection department of the local district attorney's office to see if there are any complaints against the club.
- Again, do not sign a contract on the spot. Double check what the monthly fees are and ask what the initial joining fee is.
- How do you quit the gym? Do you need to show proof of moving from the area? Do you have to pay a fee?
- Check with your insurance company. Often many insurance companies reinburse some or all of the cost of a gym membership.
- How far is the gym from your house and work? If it is too far out of the way, will you go enough to make joining the gym a cost-effective decision?

- Does the fitness professional have **CPR** certification, the appropriate educational background, and fitness certification from nationally recognized organizations? Is the fitness professional accredited?
- Does the fitness professional abide by recognized regulations, standards, or guidelines accepted for personalized training in the fitness industry, and if so, what are they?

Precautions When Using Hydrotherapy Equipment

One of the pleasures of a health club can be using the sauna, steam bath, whirlpool, or hot tub. They do not do anything to make you more fit, but they can make you feel better. However, there are some precautions to keep in mind:

- Make sure the equipment is kept clean, and that a hot tub/whirlpool is chlorinated and has the right **pH**.
- Make sure the temperature is not hotter than: 100°F for a whirlpool/hot tub; 120°F for a steam bath; 190°F for a sauna.
- Shower with soap before and after use.
- Don't stay in longer than 10–15 minutes.
- Stay hydrated: Drink water before or during use.
- Be careful about overheating yourself:
  - Wait an hour after eating.
  - Cool down after exercising.
  - Don't drink alcohol beforehand.
  - Don't exercise while you are in there.
  - Get out immediately if you get a headache, or feel dizzy, hot, chilled, or nauseated.
- Don't wear makeup, skin lotion, or jewelry.
- Don't go in by yourself.
- If you have any health problems or are on medication, check first with your doctor.
- Do not submerse you entire body if you have a heart condition or may be pregnant. The hot temperature may cause an adverse effect.

What's the word. . .

CPR (cardiopulmonary resuscitation) Clearing air passages to the lungs, giving mouth-to-mouth respiration, and massaging the heart to restore normal breathing after cardiac arrest.

pH Condition of a solution represented by a number on a scale of acidity to alkalinity.

Purchasing Exercise Equipment

After checking the advertised claims for exercise equipment, consider these questions before buying:

- Most important, will the equipment help you achieve your desired goal—build strength, improve endurance, etc.?
- Will you use the equipment? Most home exercise equipment goes unused.
- Do you have room for it?

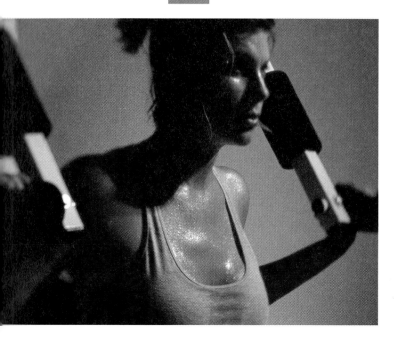

- Will you have to disassemble the equipment to store it?
- Is it so noisy it will bother your neighbors?
- Check out consumer and fitness magazines that rate exercise equipment.
- Test equipment at a local gym or retailer to find one that feels comfortable to you.
- What's the best deal? Shop around.
- Get details on warranties, guarantees, and return policies. Try to buy from a seller who offers a 30-day money-back guarantee.
- Check out the seller's customer service and support.

You may get a great deal from a secondhand store, consignment shop, yard sale, or the classified ads. But be aware:

- Items bought secondhand usually cannot be returned and don't carry the warranties of new equipment.
- Ask about total costs before buying. The ad may quote a low price, but not include shipping and handling fees, sales tax, and delivery and set-up fees.

Exercise Myths or Misconceptions

Misconceptions exist about what is exercise fact and what is exercise fiction. Here are some common exercise-related fallacies:

- Passive muscle stimulators expend energy from the electrical outlet in the wall, not from your cells. The energy expended to bring about fat loss must be from within your body.
- Taking a pill to bring about instant changes in fitness is an illusion. Fitness takes time and effort. The body systems (muscular, cardiovascular, and skeletal) become stronger in response to regular physical activity.
- **Cellulite** is not something a health gadget or cream can eliminate. Rapid gain or loss of body fat causes the dimpled look associated with the term *cellulite*.
- Shake, rattle, or roll your fat—it won't disappear. The *only* way to reduce body fat is to use more energy than you consume in calories.
- Wearing rubberized suits, extra layers of clothing, or working out in a hot environment loses water, not fat. It takes a great deal of heat to melt fat, which would melt the rest of you as well.
- If spot reduction worked, everyone who chewed gum or talked a lot would have a narrow face.
- Exercise does not turn fat cells into muscle cells, nor does inactivity turn muscle cells into fat. They are different types of cells. Eat too much and be inactive, and you will enlarge (**hypertrophy**) the fat cells in your body and shrink (**atrophy**) the muscle cells. Eat right and be physically active to do the reverse.
- Rubbing lotions on the skin to lose fat, firm up muscles, or remove lactic acid does not work. Resistance training firms up muscles.

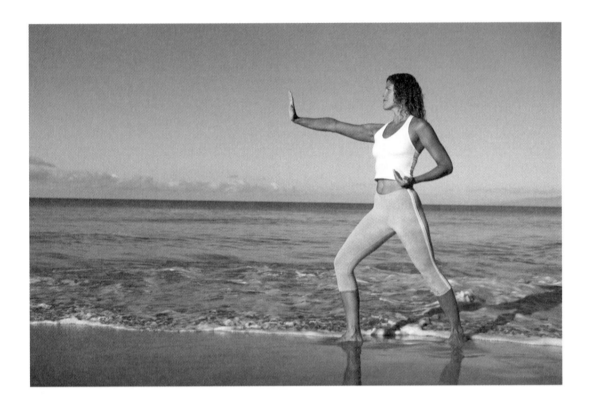

- Eating extra protein to build stronger muscles doesn't work. Eat more protein than your body uses and the extra will be stored by your body as fat. Increased muscle size comes through resistance training.
- Losing inches is not necessarily loss of fat. It can also be loss of water or lean muscle tissue.
- Exercise is only tiring momentarily. It then makes you feel more energetic as you become more fit.
- In women, resistance training mainly increases muscle strength, not size. It takes anabolic steroids (along with the training) to bulk up female bodybuilders.
- Drinking liquids during exercise does not cause cramping. Cool water or other appropriate drinks (not soda) should be drunk before, during, and after exercising to replace lost fluids.

> **What's the word. . .**
>
> **anabolic steroids** Synthetic male hormones that increase muscle size and strength.
>
> **cramping** Muscular tightness and abdominal or limb pain from dehydration and high body temperature.

Identifying Fitness Misinformation and Quackery

Some advertisers claim—without evidence—that their fitness products offer a quick, easy way to shape up, keep fit, and lose weight. There is no such thing as a no-work, no-sweat way to a healthy, fit body. To get the benefit, you have to do the work. Watch for these and other warning signs:

- If the claim sounds too good to be true, it probably is.
- If a product really worked, you would see it in headlines, not just in ads.

- The ads claim the product treats a wide range of ailments.
- The information given is unclear, vague, and highly emotional.
- Changes are promised to be quick, dramatic, or miraculous.
- Results are promised to be easy, effortless, guaranteed, or permanent.
- The ads claim relief from conditions for which there are few treatments and no cures.
- The promoter blames problems on a build-up of toxins in the body.
- Ads declare the medical community to be against the discovery.
- The ads rely on a guru, testimonials, case histories, and before-and-after photos.
- Products are sold door-to-door, in fliers, pop-up ads, or by mail order and television advertisements.
- The promoter uses high-pressure sales tactics, one-time-only deals, recruitment for a pyramid sales organization, or demands for large advance payments or long-term contracts.

Reflect ›››› Reinforce ›››› Reinvigorate

Knowledge Check

Answers in Appendix D

1. If you don't begin exercising when you are young, you will never get any benefit from it.
   A. True
   B. False
2. Perhaps the most important question to ask yourself when purchasing a piece of exercise equipment is:
   A. Do I have room for it?
   B. Will I use the equipment?
   C. Will the equipment help me achieve my goals (e.g., build strength)?
3. What should you look for in using a hot tub?
   A. It's clean.
   B. It has 12, not 6, jets.
   C. The bubbler signals you when to get out.

Modern Modifications

- Look through your local community education or college intramurals programs for a new activity or sport class that you would like to try.
- Aerobic classes or sports not your style? Learn a new type of dance instead.
- Take a walk during your lunch break.
- Ride a bike or walk to work or class if you live a reasonable distance away.
- Check any supplements or home exercise equipment that you have at home using the guidelines provided in this chapter.

Conclusion

After reading this book, and especially this chapter, you should realize that many decisions are necessary for maintaining a healthy lifestyle. To make good decisions, you can use the following procedure. This procedure applies to any of life's decisions, not merely those dealing with a healthy lifestyle.

1. Identify and clarify the problem. You must recognize that a problem exists. Some may simply be annoyances, while others are big issues.
2. Gather information. Learn more about the problem situation. Look for possible causes and solutions.
3. Evaluate the evidence. How accurate is the information? Is it fact or opinion?
4. Consider alternatives and implications. Draw conclusions, then weigh the advantages and disadvantages of each alternative.
5. Choose and implement the best alternative.

Use a log to keep track of your progress from week to week, month to month, and year to year for any one of the healthy lifestyle behaviors you are pursuing.

Critical Thinking

Answers in Appendix D

Scenario One: Phil is a 55-year-old overweight salesman with high blood pressure. What course of action do you recommend to help him reach his 56th birthday?

A. He should immediately join a gym and start vigorous daily workouts.
B. He should check with his doctor about starting a program of gradually increasing daily physical activity coupled with a better diet.
C. He should cut down a bit on the martinis at lunch.
D. He doesn't need to change anything so long as he feels OK.

Scenario Two: Sales of health and fitness club memberships are at an all-time high. What should you do in selecting a health/fitness club for your workouts?

A. Ask questions (e.g., What are the trainers' credentials?).
B. Check out the social amenities the club offers.
C. Look around to see if everyone in the club looks fit.
D. All of the above.

Scenario Three: Your mother has Alzheimer's. You want to help her in every way possible. In a magazine you read this advertisement: "Cure Alzheimer's Disease!!! My husband has Alzheimer's. On September 2, 1998, he began taking one teaspoon a day of Emu's Liver Oil. Now (in just 22 days) he mows the grass, cleans out the garage, weeds the flower beds, and we take our morning walk again. It hasn't helped his memory much yet, but he is more like himself!!!" What sends a warning signal that this product and its claims may not be valid?

A. The ad appeared in a magazine.
B. An unsupported testimonial is used to sell the product.
C. Emus do not develop Alzheimer's.

Going Above and Beyond
Websites
American Dietetics Association
http://www.eatright.org

American Medical Association, Health Insight
http://www.ama-assn.org

Center for Science in the Public Interest
http://www.cspinet.org

Food and Drug Administration
http://www.fda.gov

Healthfinder
http://www.healthfinder.gov

Mayo Clinic
http://www.mayohealth.org

National Council Against Health Fraud
http://www.ncahf.org

National Council for Reliable Health Information
http://www.ncahf.org

Office of Dietary Supplements
http://dietarysupplements.info.nih.gov

Quackwatch
http://quackwatch.com

References and Suggested Readings

Angell M. and Kassirer J. P. Alternative medicine: The risks of untested and unregulated remedies. *New England Journal of Medicine* 339(12)(1998):839.

Armsey T. D. and Gree G. A. Nutrition supplements: Science vs. hype. *Physician and Sports Medicine* 25(6)(1997):76.

The mainstreaming of alternative medicine. *Consumer Reports* 65(5)(2000):17–25.

Kuntzleman C. T. and Wilkerson R. A primer to recommending home aerobic equipment. *American College of Sports Medicine Health and Fitness Journal* 1(6)(1997):24.

Stamford B. Choosing and using exercise equipment. *Physician and Sports Medicine* 25(1)(1997):107–108.

Dietary Guidelines for Americans 2005*

The *Dietary Guidelines for Americans* provides science-based advice to promote health and to reduce risk for major chronic diseases through diet and physical activity. Major causes of morbidity and mortality in the United States are related to poor diet and a sedentary lifestyle. Some specific diseases linked to poor diet and physical inactivity include cardiovascular disease, type 2 diabetes, hypertension, osteoporosis, and certain cancers. Furthermore, poor diet and physical inactivity, resulting in an energy imbalance (more calories consumed than expended), are the most important factors contributing to the increase in overweight and obesity in this country. Combined with physical activity, following a diet that does not provide excess calories according to the recommendations in this document should enhance the health of most individuals.

Adequate Nutrients within Calorie Needs

Key Recommendations

- Consume a variety of nutrient-dense foods and beverages within and among the basic food groups while choosing foods that limit the intake of saturated and *trans* fats, cholesterol, added sugars, salt, and alcohol.
- Meet recommended intakes within energy needs by adopting a balanced eating pattern, such as the USDA Food Guide or the DASH Eating Plan.

Key Recommendations for Specific Population Groups

- *People over age 50.* Consume vitamin B_{12} in its crystalline form (i.e., fortified foods or supplements).
- *Women of childbearing age who may become pregnant.* Eat foods high in heme-iron and/or consume iron-rich plant foods or iron-fortified foods with an enhancer of iron absorption, such as vitamin C-rich foods.
- *Women of childbearing age who may become pregnant and those in the first trimester of pregnancy.* Consume adequate synthetic folic acid daily (from fortified foods or supplements) in addition to food forms of folate from a varied diet.
- *Older adults, people with dark skin, and people exposed to insufficient ultraviolet band radiation (i.e., sunlight).* Consume extra vitamin D from vitamin D-fortified foods and/or supplements.

Weight Management

Key Recommendations

- To maintain body weight in a healthy range, balance calories from foods and beverages with calories expended.

*From Department of Health and Human Services (HHS) and the Department of Agriculture (USDA), *Dietary Guidelines for Americans 2005*, joint statement released on January 12, 2005. http://www.healthierus.gov/dietaryguidelines/.

A

- To prevent gradual weight gain over time, make small decreases in food and beverage calories and increase physical activity.

Key Recommendations for Specific Population Groups

- *Those who need to lose weight.* Aim for a slow, steady weight loss by decreasing calorie intake while maintaining an adequate nutrient intake and increasing physical activity.
- *Overweight children.* Reduce the rate of body weight gain while allowing growth and development. Consult a healthcare provider before placing a child on a weight-reduction diet.
- *Pregnant women.* Ensure appropriate weight gain as specified by a healthcare provider.
- *Breastfeeding women.* Moderate weight reduction is safe and does not compromise weight gain of the nursing infant.
- *Overweight adults and overweight children with chronic diseases and/or on medication.* Consult a healthcare provider about weight loss strategies prior to starting a weight-reduction program to ensure appropriate management of other health conditions.

Physical Activity

Key Recommendations

- Engage in regular physical activity and reduce sedentary activities to promote health, psychological well-being, and a healthy body weight.
  - To reduce the risk of chronic disease in adulthood: Engage in at least 30 minutes of moderate-intensity physical activity, above usual activity, at work or home on most days of the week.
  - For most people, greater health benefits can be obtained by engaging in physical activity of more vigorous intensity or longer duration.
  - To help manage body weight and prevent gradual, unhealthy body weight gain in adulthood: Engage in approximately 60 minutes of moderate- to vigorous-intensity activity on most days of the week while not exceeding caloric intake requirements.
  - To sustain weight loss in adulthood: Participate in at least 60 to 90 minutes of daily moderate-intensity physical activity while not exceeding caloric intake requirements. Some people may need to consult with a healthcare provider before participating in this level of activity.
- Achieve physical fitness by including cardiovascular conditioning, stretching exercises for flexibility, and resistance exercises or calisthenics for muscle strength and endurance.

Key Recommendations for Specific Population Groups

- *Children and adolescents.* Engage in at least 60 minutes of physical activity on most, preferably all, days of the week.
- *Pregnant women.* In the absence of medical or obstetric complications, incorporate 30 minutes or more of moderate-intensity physical activity on most, if not all, days of the week. Avoid activities with a high risk of falling or abdominal trauma.
- *Breastfeeding women.* Be aware that neither acute nor regular exercise adversely affects the mother's ability to successfully breastfeed.

- *Older adults.* Participate in regular physical activity to reduce functional declines associated with aging and to achieve the other benefits of physical activity identified for all adults.

Food Groups to Encourage

Key Recommendations

- Consume a sufficient amount of fruits and vegetables while staying within energy needs. Two cups of fruit and 2½ cups of vegetables per day are recommended for a reference 2,000-calorie intake, with higher or lower amounts depending on the calorie level.
- Choose a variety of fruits and vegetables each day. In particular, select from all five vegetable subgroups (dark green, orange, legumes, starchy vegetables, and other vegetables) several times a week.
- Consume 3 or more ounce-equivalents of whole-grain products per day, with the rest of the recommended grains coming from enriched or whole-grain products. In general, at least half the grains should come from whole grains.
- Consume 3 cups per day of fat-free or low-fat milk or equivalent milk products.

Key Recommendations for Specific Population Groups

- *Children and adolescents.* Consume whole-grain products often; at least half the grains should be whole grains. Children 2 to 8 years should consume 2 cups per day of fat-free or low-fat milk or equivalent milk products. Children 9 years of age and older should consume 3 cups per day of fat-free or low-fat milk or equivalent milk products.

Fats

Key Recommendations

- Consume less than 10 percent of calories from saturated fatty acids and less than 300 mg/day of cholesterol, and keep *trans* fatty acid consumption as low as possible.
- Keep total fat intake between 20 to 35 percent of calories, with most fats coming from sources of polyunsaturated and monounsaturated fatty acids, such as fish, nuts, and vegetable oils.
- When selecting and preparing meat, poultry, dry beans, and milk or milk products, make choices that are lean, low-fat, or fat-free.
- Limit intake of fats and oils high in saturated and/or *trans* fatty acids, and choose products low in such fats and oils.

Key Recommendations for Specific Population Groups

- *Children and adolescents.* Keep total fat intake between 30 to 35 percent of calories for children 2 to 3 years of age and between 25 to 35 percent of calories for children and adolescents 4 to 18 years of age, with most fats coming from sources of polyunsaturated and monounsaturated fatty acids, such as fish, nuts, and vegetable oils.

Carbohydrates

Key Recommendations

- Choose fiber-rich fruits, vegetables, and whole grains often.
- Choose and prepare foods and beverages with little added sugars or caloric sweeteners, such as amounts suggested by the USDA Food Guide and the DASH Eating Plan.
- Reduce the incidence of dental caries by practicing good oral hygiene and consuming sugar- and starch-containing foods and beverages less frequently.

Sodium and Potassium

Key Recommendations

- Consume less than 2,300 mg (approximately 1 tsp of salt) of sodium per day.
- Choose and prepare foods with little salt. At the same time, consume potassium-rich foods, such as fruits and vegetables.

Key Recommendations for Specific Population Groups

- *Individuals with hypertension, blacks, and middle-aged and older adults.* Aim to consume no more than 1,500 mg of sodium per day, and meet the potassium recommendation (4,700 mg/day) with food.

Alcoholic Beverages

Key Recommendations

- Those who choose to drink alcoholic beverages should do so sensibly and in moderation—defined as the consumption of up to one drink per day for women and up to two drinks per day for men.
- Alcoholic beverages should not be consumed by some individuals, including those who cannot restrict their alcohol intake, women of childbearing age who may become pregnant, pregnant and lactating women, children and adolescents, individuals taking medications that can interact with alcohol, and those with specific medical conditions.
- Alcoholic beverages should be avoided by individuals engaging in activities that require attention, skill, or coordination, such as driving or operating machinery.

Food Safety

Key Recommendations

- To avoid microbial foodborne illness:
  - Clean hands, food contact surfaces, and fruits and vegetables. Meat and poultry should not be washed or rinsed.
  - Separate raw, cooked, and ready-to-eat foods while shopping, preparing, or storing foods.
  - Cook foods to a safe temperature to kill microorganisms.

- Chill (refrigerate) perishable food promptly and defrost foods properly.
- Avoid raw (unpasteurized) milk or any products made from unpasteurized milk, raw or partially cooked eggs or foods containing raw eggs, raw or undercooked meat and poultry, unpasteurized juices, and raw sprouts.

Key Recommendations for Specific Population Groups

- *Infants and young children, pregnant women, older adults, and those who are immuno-compromised.* Do not eat or drink raw (unpasteurized) milk or any products made from unpasteurized milk, raw or partially cooked eggs or foods containing raw eggs, raw or undercooked meat and poultry, raw or undercooked fish or shellfish, unpasteurized juices, and raw sprouts.
- *Pregnant women, older adults, and those who are immunocompromised:* Only eat certain deli meats and frankfurters that have been reheated to steaming hot.

Nutrition and Health for Canadians*

Canadian Guidelines for Nutrition

For the past 60 years, the government has worked to promote healthy and nutritious eating habits in Canadians. In 1987, Health and Welfare Canada began a major review of the system for guiding Canadians on their food choices. To perform the review, the government appointed two advisory committees—the Scientific Review Committee and the Communications and Implementation Committee.

After examining research evidence available on nutrition and public health, the Scientific Review Committee issued a report in 1990 called Nutrition Recommendations. The report included both updated Recommended Nutrient Intakes (RNI) and a scientific description of a healthy dietary pattern that would deliver adequate nutrients for health and reduce the risk of nutrition-related chronic diseases.

Meanwhile, the Communications and Implementation Committee translated these scientific findings into understandable guidelines and outlined implementation strategies in a report called *Action Towards Healthy Eating: Technical Report* (1990). This report suggested that Canada develop a "total diet approach" towards healthy eating. A total diet approach would give consumers a better idea of eating patterns associated with reducing the risk of developing chronic diseases.

In 1990, the government issued *Nutrition Recommendations: A Call for Action*, a summary report produced jointly by the Scientific Review Committee and the Communications and Implementation Committee.

A Revised Food Guide

In accordance with the recommendations of its two advisory groups, the Health Department undertook to revise *Canada's Food Guide*. In 1992, the agency launched *Canada's Food Guide to Healthy Eating* and an explanatory document called *Using the Food Guide*. This promotes dietary diversity, reducing total fat intake, and an active lifestyle. It also offers consumers a pattern for establishing healthy eating habits in their daily selection of foods.

Moreover, the guide introduced a number of new concepts. A range of servings from the four food groups accommodates the wide range of energy needs for different ages, body sizes, activity levels, genders, and conditions such as pregnancy and nursing. The wide range of servings in grain products, vegetables, and fruits is designed to give consumers a better idea of the type of diet that would help reduce the risk of developing nutrition-related chronic diseases.

The guide also introduced a category of "other" foods such as sweets, fats such as butter, and drinks like coffee that, though part of the diets of many Canadians, would traditionally not have been mentioned in a food guide. The guide recommends moderation in the consumption of these foods and acknowledges their role, along with the wide range of servings in grains, vegetables, and fruits, as a "total diet approach" to healthy eating.

*Adapted with permission from Insel, P., Turner, R.E., and Ross, D. *Nutrition*, 2nd ed. Sudbury, MA: Jones and Bartlett Publishers, 2004.

A Work in Progress

Some groups and organizations challenged specific aspects of the government's Nutrition Recommendations. In a typically Canadian twist, the government responded to challengers by including them in the development process. When the Canadian Pediatric Society, for example, queried the dietary recommendations on fat consumption in children, the Society was invited to join Health Canada in researching the issue. The result was *Nutrition Recommendations Update: Dietary Fat and Children* (1993), which adjusted the recommendation of appropriate levels of dietary fat for growing children. In 1995, Health Canada issued *Canada's Food Guide to Healthy Eating: Focus on Preschoolers* as a background paper for educators and communicators.

Health Canada also has positioned nutrition in a broader health context, which includes physical activity and a positive outlook on life. One result of this comprehensive approach was the *Vitality Leaders Kit* (1994), intended to help community leaders promote healthy eating, active living, and positive self- and body-image in an integrated way.

Canada's *Food Guide to Healthy Eating*

Scientists have known for some time that adequate nutrition is essential for proper growth and development. More recently, healthy eating has been accepted as a significant factor in reducing the risk of developing nutrition-related problems, including heart disease, cancer, obesity, hypertension (high blood pressure), osteoporosis, anemia, dental decay, and some bowel disorders.

Healthy Eating in Canada

The Food Guide is based on nutrition and food science. A key reference is *Nutrition Recommendations: The Report of the Scientific Review Committee*, published in 1990 by Health Canada. This report contains a review of nutrition research conducted by a committee of scientists and provides recommendations describing the desired characteristics of the Canadian diet. The Nutrition Recommendations, which are reviewed regularly, act as the foundation for all nutrition and healthy eating programs in the country.

Canada's Guidelines for Healthy Eating

A committee of experts in communications and program planning worked with the committee of scientists and prepared the report *Action Towards Healthy Eating*. They adapted the Nutrition Recommendations into a more user-friendly set of statements called *Canada's Guidelines for Healthy Eating*. These Guidelines promote healthy eating in a general way:

- Enjoy a variety of foods.
- Emphasize cereals, breads, other grain products, vegetables, and fruit.
- Choose lower-fat dairy products, leaner meats, and foods prepared with little or no fat.
- Achieve and maintain a healthy body weight by enjoying regular physical activity and healthy eating.
- Limit salt, alcohol, and caffeine.

Canada's Food Guide to Healthy Eating

Canada's Food Guide to Healthy Eating takes *Canada's Guidelines for Healthy Eating* one step further and provides consumers with more detailed information for establishing healthy eating habits through the daily selection of food ⬤ **Figure B.1** . The Food Guide is a basic nutrition education tool used:

- to help plan healthy meals for individuals or groups; and
- to evaluate a person's eating habits in a general way but not to assess nutritional status.

The Food Guide meets the nutritional needs of all Canadians four years of age and over and has been designed specifically for the general public with a reading level of grade seven. It is not appropriate for those under the age of four because the number of servings and the serving sizes are too large for toddlers and preschoolers.

Food Guide Materials

- *Canada's Food Guide to Healthy Eating*: a tear sheet for consumers.
- *Using the Food Guide*: a booklet for consumers that explains the basic concepts of the tear sheet more fully.
- *Food Guide Facts*: Background for Educators and Communicators: fact sheets that provide background information for nutrition professionals, health educators, home economists, fitness leaders, and others involved in promoting healthy eating.
- *Canada's Food Guide to Healthy Eating*: tear sheet, consumer booklet and the fact sheets for educators and communicators are available from provincial or local health departments or from: Publications, Health Canada, Ottawa, Ontario K1A 0K9, tel. (613) 954-5995.

Canada's Physical Activity Guide to Healthy Active Living

High levels of physical inactivity are a serious threat to public health in Canada. Nearly two-thirds of Canadians are not active enough to achieve optimal health benefits. These Canadians are at risk for heart disease, obesity, high blood pressure, adult-onset diabetes, osteoporosis, stroke, depression, and colon cancer. Although physical activity levels increased during the 1980s and early 1990s, the progress has stalled. Health Canada estimates that physical inactivity results in at least 21,000 premature deaths annually.

Canada's Physical Activity Guide to Healthy Active Living, produced by a joint effort of Health Canada and the Canadian Society for Exercise Physiology, provides the first set of Canadian guidelines for physical activity ⬤ **Figure B.2** . It provides information to help Canadians understand how to achieve health benefits by being physically active. The guide complements the popular *Canada's Food Guide to Healthy Eating* and provides concrete examples of how to incorporate physical activity into daily life.

Designed for adults, the guide recommends 60 minutes of physical activity every day to stay healthy or improve your health. As a person progresses to more intense activity, they can cut down to 30 minutes, four days a week. The guide also suggests Canadians can add up their activities in periods of at least 10 minutes each, starting slowly and building up.

Federal, provincial, and territorial governments are working to reduce the number of inactive Canadians. *Canada's Physical Activity Guide to Healthy Active Living* is a major step toward building the knowledge and awareness necessary for all Canadians to become more active. The healthy active living series now also includes *Physical Activity Guide to Healthy Active Living for Older Adults*, *Physical Activity Guide for Youth*, *Physical Activity Guide for Children*, and *Active Living at Work*.

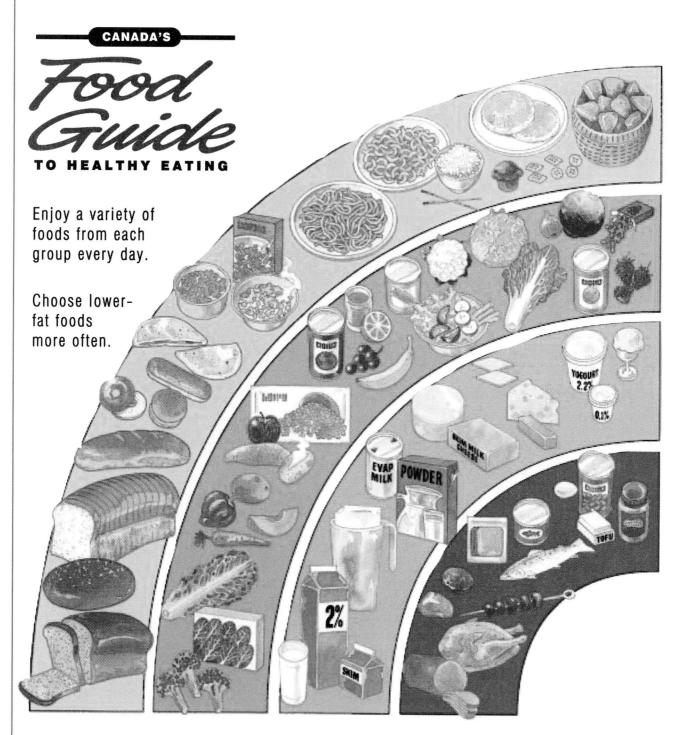

CANADA'S

Food Guide
TO HEALTHY EATING

Enjoy a variety of foods from each group every day.

Choose lower-fat foods more often.

Grain Products
Choose whole grain and enriched products more often

Vegetables & Fruit
Choose dark green and orange vegetables and orange fruit more often.

Milk Products
Choose lower-fat milk products more often

Meat & Alternatives
Choose leaner meats, poultry and fish, as well as dried peas, beans and lentils more often

Figure B.1

Canada's Food Guide. Source: © Minister of Public Works and Government Services Canada, 1997.

Different People Need Different Amounts of Food

The amount of food you need every day from the 4 groups and other foods depends on your age, body size, activity level, whether you are male or female and if you are pregnant or breast-feeding. That's why the Food Guide gives a lower and higher number of servings for each food group. For example, young children can choose the number of servings, while male teenagers can go to the higher number. Most other people can choose servings somewhere in between.

Grain Products
5–12
SERVINGS PER DAY

Vegetables and Fruit
5–10
SERVINGS PER DAY

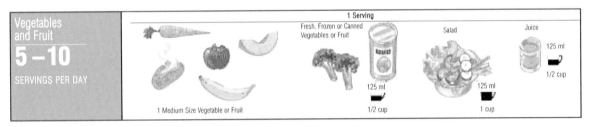

Milk Products
SERVINGS PER DAY
Children 4–9 years: 2–3
Youth 10–16 years: 3–4
Adults: 2–4
Pregnant and Breast-feeding Women 3–4

Other Foods

Taste and enjoyment can also come from other foods and beverages that are not part of the 4 food groups. Some of these foods are higher in fat or calories, so use these foods in moderation.

Meat and Alternatives
2–3
SERVINGS PER DAY

Enjoy eating well, being active and feeling good about yourself. That's *VITALITé*

©Minister of Supply and Services Canada 1992 Cat. No. H39-252/1992E No changes permitted. Reprint permission not required.
ISBN 0-662-19648-1

Health Canada   Santé Canada

 Canadian Society for Exercise Physiology

Figure B.2

Canada's Physical Activity Guide. Source: © Minister of Public Works and Government Services Canada, 1997.

Choose a variety of activities from these three groups:

Endurance

4 - 7 days a week
Continuous activities for your heart, lungs and circulatory system.

Flexibility

4 - 7 days a week
Gentle reaching, bending and stretching activities to keep your muscles relaxed and joints mobile.

Strength

2 - 4 days a week
Activities against resistance to strengthen muscles and bones and improve posture.

Starting slowly is very safe for most people. Not sure? Consult your health professional.

For a copy of the *Guide Handbook* and more information:
1-888-334-9769, or **www.paguide.com**

Eating well is also important. Follow *Canada's Food Guide to Healthy Eating* to make wise food choices.

Get Active Your Way, Every Day—For Life!

Scientists say accumulate 60 minutes of physical activity every day to stay healthy or improve your health. As you progress to moderate activities you can cut down to 30 minutes, 4 days a week. Add-up your activities in periods of at least 10 minutes each. Start slowly... and build up.

Time needed depends on effort

Very Light Effort	Light Effort *60 minutes*	Moderate Effort *30 - 60 minutes*	Vigorous Effort *20 - 30 minutes*	Maximum Effort
• Strolling • Dusting	• Light walking • Volleyball • Easy gardening • Stretching	• Brisk walking • Biking • Raking leaves • Swimming • Dancing • Water aerobics	• Aerobics • Jogging • Hockey • Basketball • Fast swimming • Fast dancing	• Sprinting • Racing

Range needed to stay healthy

You Can Do It – Getting started is easier than you think

Physical activity doesn't have to be very hard. Build physical activities into your daily routine.

- Walk whenever you can – get off the bus early, use the stairs instead of the elevator.
- Reduce inactivity for long periods, like watching TV.
- Get up from the couch and stretch and bend for a few minutes every hour.
- Play actively with your kids.
- Choose to walk, wheel or cycle for short trips.

- Start with a 10 minute walk – gradually increase the time.
- Find out about walking and cycling paths nearby and use them.
- Observe a physical activity class to see if you want to try it.
- Try one class to start – you don't have to make a long-term commitment.
- Do the activities you are doing now, more often.

Benefits of regular activity:	Health risks of inactivity:
• better health • improved fitness • better posture and balance • better self-esteem • weight control • stronger muscles and bones • feeling more energetic • relaxation and reduced stress • continued independent living in later life	• premature death • heart disease • obesity • high blood pressure • adult-onset diabetes • osteoporosis • stroke • depression • colon cancer

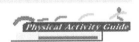

B

Nutrition Labeling for Canadians

The nutrition label is one of the most useful tools in selecting foods for healthy eating. The Food Guide outlines a pattern of healthy eating; the nutrition label supports the Food Guide by helping consumers to choose foods according to healthy eating messages.

Consumers can use labels to compare products and make choices on the basis of nutrient content. For example, consumers can choose a lower-fat product based on the fat content given on the labels **Figure B.3** and **Figure B.4**.

Consumers also can use label information to evaluate products in relation to healthy eating. For instance, the Nutrition Recommendations advise Canadians to get 30 percent or less of their day's energy (kilocalories/kilojoules) from fat. This translates into a range of fat, in grams, that can be used as a benchmark against which individual foods and meals can be evaluated. The Food Guide covers a range of energy needs from 1,800 to 3,200 kilocalories (7,500 to 13,400 kilojoules) per day. A fat intake of 30 percent or less of a day's calories means a fat intake between 60 and 105 grams of fat.

Label Claims

A claim on a food label highlights a nutritional feature of a product. It is known to influence consumers' buying habits. Manufacturers often position label claims in a bold, banner-format on the front panel of a package or on the side panel along with the nutrition label. Since a label claim must be backed up by detailed facts relating to the claim, the consumer should look for the nutrition label for more information.

Nutrient Content Claims

A nutrient content claim describes the amount of a nutrient in a food. A food whose label carries the claim high fibre must contain 4 grams or more fibre per reference amount and serving of stated size. A "sodium-free" food must contain less than 5 mg of sodium per reference amount and serving of stated size.

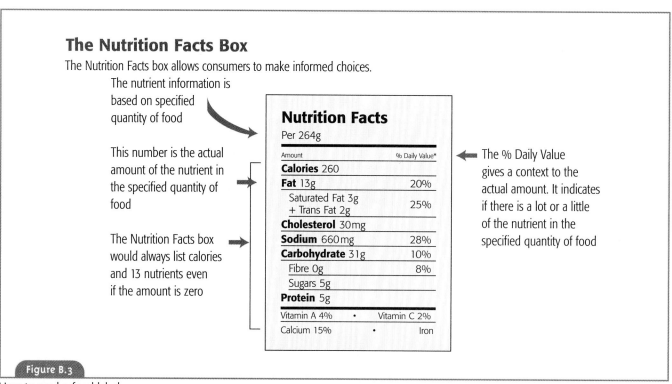

The Nutrition Facts Box

The Nutrition Facts box allows consumers to make informed choices.

The nutrient information is based on specified quantity of food

This number is the actual amount of the nutrient in the specified quantity of food

The Nutrition Facts box would always list calories and 13 nutrients even if the amount is zero

Nutrition Facts
Per 264g

Amount	% Daily Value*
Calories 260	
Fat 13g	20%
Saturated Fat 3g + Trans Fat 2g	25%
Cholesterol 30mg	
Sodium 660mg	28%
Carbohydrate 31g	10%
Fibre 0g	8%
Sugars 5g	
Protein 5g	
Vitamin A 4% • Vitamin C 2%	
Calcium 15% • Iron	

The % Daily Value gives a context to the actual amount. It indicates if there is a lot or a little of the nutrient in the specified quantity of food

Figure B.3

How to read a food label.

INGREDIENTS: Fructose Syrup (from Grapes, Corn and Pears), Oat Bran, Maltodextrin (Complex Carbohydrate), Modified Milk Ingredients (Milk Protein with Lactose removed), Brown Rice, Almond Butter, Natural Berry Flavours, Carmine, Citric Acid, **VITAMINS AND MINERALS:** Dicalcium phosphate, Potassium bicarbonate, Ascorbic acid, Magnesium carbonate, Alpha tocopherol (vit. E), Zinc gluconate, Ferrous fumarate, Salt, Potassium iodide, Beta carotene (vit. A), Copper gluconate, Manganese sulfate, Calcium pantothenate, Pyridoxine hydrochloride (vit. B_6), Riboflavin (vit B_2), Niacin, Thiamin hydrochloride (vit. B_1), Cholecalciferol (vit. D), Folic acid, Biotin, Cyanocobalamin (vit. B_{12}).

INGRÉDIENTS: Sirop de fructose (de Raisin, de Maïs et de Poire), Son d'avione, Maltodextrine (glucide complexe), Substances latières modifées (protéines du lait, lactose enlevé), Riz brun, Beurre d'amande, Arômes naturels de baie, Carmin, Acide citrique, **VITAMINES ET MINERAUX:** Phosphate bicalcique, Bicarbonate de potassium, Acide ascorbique, Carbonate de magnésium, Alpha tocophérol (vit. E), Gluconate de zinc Fumarate ferreux, Sel, Iodure de potassium, Bêta-carotène (vit. A), Gluconate de cuivre, Sulfate de manganèse, Pantothénate de calcium, Chlorhydrate de pyridoxine (vit. B_6) Riboflavine (vit. B_2), Niacine, Chlorhydrate de thiamine (vit. B_1) Cholécalciférol (vit. D), Acide folique, Biotine, Cyanocobalamine (vit. B_{12}).

Ingredients List must be included by law and must list all of the ingredients used in the product. Ingredients are listed in the order of the amount used. The amount is based on the weight of an ingredient rather than its volume.

Figure B.4

Ingredients list.

Diet-Related Health Claims

Optional health claims highlight the characteristics of a diet that reduces the chance of developing a disease such as cancer or heart disease. They also tell how the food fits into the diet.

Characteristic of the Diet:	Reduced Risk of:
Low in sodium and high in potassium	High blood pressure
Adequate in calcium and vitamin D	Osteoporosis
Low in saturated and trans fats	Heart disease
Rich in fruit and vegetables	Some types of cancer
Sugar alcohols (such as sorbitol)	Tooth decay

New nutrition labeling regulations were published on January 1, 2003. For the latest information, visit the Nutrition Labeling area of the Health Canada Web site at: http://www.hc-sc.gc.ca/hpfb-dgpsa/onpp-bppn/labelling-etiquetage/index_e.html.

Food Choice System

The CDA Food Choice System is a method of meal planning created by the Canadian Diabetes Association to make it easier for people with diabetes to eat the right amount of food for their insulin supply. This system is based on two concepts: Most foods are eaten by people with diabetes in measured amounts, and foods within each of the system's seven food groups can be interchanged.

The CDA Food Choice System started with the nutritional principles in *Canada's Food Guide to Healthy Eating* and modified them to meet the special needs of people with dia-

B

betes. People with diabetes must eat a certain amount of carbohydrate, protein, and fat at each meal in order to control the amount of glucose (sugar) that enters the blood after a meal. The CDA Food Choice System helps them select the proper type and amount of food to manage their diabetes.

The Food Choice System classifies foods into seven food groups according to the food's carbohydrate, protein, and fat content. The Food Choice Values tell a person with diabetes what group a food belongs to and how much of that food is interchangeable with another food in the same food group. The Food Choice Values, therefore, help someone with diabetes eat a balance of foods in the right amounts.

In the Food Choice System, the seven food groups and their symbols are:

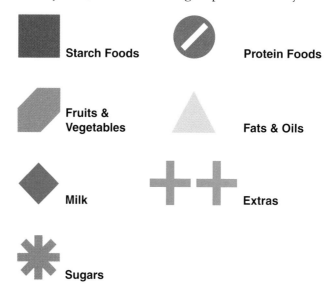

Because food groups in CDA's Food Choice Systems may be confused with the food groups in *Canada's Food Guide to Healthy Eating*, the government does not permit them to be listed by name on food labels. The Federal government regulation states that only the assigned quantity, the Food Choice "Symbol," and the word "Choice" can be published on a label.

Injury Care and Prevention

Exercise-Related Injuries

Most exercise-related injuries do not threaten life, nor are they severe. However, exercise-related injuries demand that you make a decision about the proper care for an injury.

This section helps in such decision-making with its decision-table (If…, then…) format. Decision tables not only help identify what may be wrong (the "If" column), but also help determine what action to take (the "Then" column).

This section does not cover life-threatening conditions requiring rescue breathing and CPR, nor many other injuries and conditions that a quality first aid course may cover. For a quality first aid course, go to the American Academy of Orthopaedic Surgeons/American College of Emergency Physicians Emergency Care and Safety Institute website— http://www.safetycampus.org—to locate a training center near you. Many colleges and universities use the AAOS/ACEP first aid, CPR, and AED (automated external defibrillator) program.

How to Examine for an Injury

See ⬤ Table C.1 ⬤.

Signs of an exercise-related injury may include:
- Loss of use. "Guarding" occurs when movement produces pain; the person refuses to use the injured part.
- A grating sensation (crepitus) can be felt, and sometimes even heard, when the ends of a broken bone rub together.

Table C.1	How to Examine for an Injury
What to Do	**How to Do It**
Determine the location of the problem.	Ask yourself or the injured person "What's wrong?" or "Where do you hurt?"
Find out if an injury exists.	Look and feel the area for one or more of the following signs of injury: deformity, open wounds, tenderness, and swelling. The mnemonic "D-O-T-S" helps in remembering the signs of an injury: • **D**eformities occur when bones are broken, causing an abnormal shape. Deformity might not be obvious. Compare the injured part with the uninjured part on the other side of the body. • **O**pen wounds break the skin and there is bleeding. • **T**enderness (pain) means sensitive when touched or pressed. It is commonly found only at the injury site. The person usually will be able to point to the site of the pain. • **S**welling is the body's response to injury that makes the area larger than usual. It appears later and is due to fluid from inflammation and/or bleeding.

For extremity (arms and legs) injuries, check blood flow and nerves. Use the mnemonic CSM (circulation, sensation, movement) as a way of remembering what to do.

- **Circulation:** For an arm injury, feel for the radial pulse (located on the thumb side of the wrist). For a leg injury, feel for the posterior tibial pulse (located between the inside ankle bone and the Achilles tendon). An arm or leg without a pulse requires immediate surgical care.
- **Sensation:** Lightly touch or squeeze one of the victim's fingers or toes and ask the victim what he or she feels. Loss of sensation is an early sign of nerve damage.
- **Movement:** Inability to move develops later. Check for nerve damage by asking the victim to wiggle his or her fingers or toes. If the fingers or toes are injured, do not have the victim try to move them.

A quick nerve and circulatory check is very important. The tissues of the arms and legs cannot survive for more than 3 hours without a continuous blood supply. If you note any disruption in the nerve and blood supply, seek immediate medical care.

RICE Procedures

RICE is the acronym—rest, ice, compression, and elevation—for the treatment of all bone, joint, and muscle injuries. The steps taken in the first 48 to 72 hours after such an injury can help to relieve, and even prevent, aches and pains.

Treat all extremity bone, joint, and muscle injuries with the RICE procedures. In addition to RICE, fractures and dislocations should be stabilized against movement.

R: Rest

Injuries heal faster if rested. Rest means to stay off the injured part and avoid moving it. Using any part of the body increases the blood circulation to that area, which can cause more swelling of an injured part.

I: Ice

An ice pack should be applied to the injured area for 20 to 30 minutes every 2 or 3 hours during the first 24 to 48 hours. Skin treated with cold passes through four stages: cold, burning, aching, and numbness. When the skin becomes numb, usually in 20 to 30 minutes, remove the ice pack. After removing the ice pack, compress the injured part with an elastic bandage and keep it elevated (the "C" and "E" of RICE).

Cold constricts the blood vessels to and in the injured area, which helps reduce the swelling and inflammation. Cold should be applied as soon as possible after the injury—healing time often is directly related to the amount of swelling that occurs. Heat has the opposite effect when applied to fresh injures: It increases circulation to the area and greatly increases both the swelling and the pain.

Put crushed ice (or cubes) into a double plastic bag or commercial ice bag. Place the ice pack directly on the skin and then use an elastic bandage to hold the ice pack in place. Ice bags can conform to the body's contours.

C: Compression

Compressing the injured area may squeeze some fluid and debris out of the injury site. Compression limits the ability of the skin and of other tissues to expand and reduces internal bleeding. Apply an elastic bandage to the injured area, especially the foot, ankle, knee, thigh, hand, or elbow. Fill the hollow areas with padding, such as a sock or washcloth, before applying the elastic bandage.

Start the elastic bandage several inches below the injury and wrap in an upward, overlapping spiral with an even, slightly tight pressure. Pale skin, pain, numbness, and tingling are signs that the bandage is too tight. If any of these appear, immediately remove the elastic bandage. Rewrap later when the symptoms disappear.

For a bruise or strain, place a pad between the injury and the elastic bandage.

E: Elevation

Elevating the injured area, in combination with ice and compression, limits circulation to an area, helps limit internal bleeding, and minimizes swelling.

Returning to Physical Activity After an Injury

Returning to physical activity is generally permissible once an injury is fully healed. Fully healed means:

- No pain
- No swelling
- No limping, favoring, or instability

Full rehabilitation means:

- Return of full range of motion and flexibility
- Muscle strength and endurance in the affected extremity (arm or leg) equal to that of the unaffected extremity
- Resumption of pre-injury endurance levels
- Good balance and coordination

Sometimes, clearance to return to exercising should come from a physician (e.g., after surgery).

Definition

- **Contusions:** Bruising of tissue.
- **Strains:** Muscles are stretched or torn.
- **Sprains:** Tearing or stretching of the joints that causes mild to severe damage to the ligaments and joint capsules.
- **Dislocations:** Bones are displaced from their normal joint alignment, out of their sockets, or out of their normal positions.
- **Tendinitis:** Inflammation of a tendon from overuse.

Specific Injuries

Foot

Foot injuries are common among exercisers because of the foot's role in bearing weight. Careless treatment can have consequences that may include lifelong disability Table C.2 .

Ankle

Most ankle injuries are sprains. About 85% of sprains involve the ankle's outside (lateral) ligaments and are caused by having the foot turned or twisted inward. If not treated properly, a sprained ankle becomes chronically susceptible for future injuries. See Table C.3 for symptoms and treatment.

Lower Leg

The two bones of the lower leg are the tibia ("shin bone") and fibula. Most shin injuries are "shin splints," which are strains from overuse. Occasionally, a bone is fractured from overuse. See Table C.4 .

Table C.2 — Determining and Treating Foot Injuries

If...	Then...
Pain is at top of the heel (over Achilles tendon) Pain is aggravated by activity—worse at beginning of activity and improved with warm-up	Suspect **Achilles tendonitis:** • Apply ice to decrease inflammation and pain. • Use an anti-inflammatory for 7 to 10 days. • Reduce or stop activity until no more pain occurs while either walking or rest. • Elevate heel with a heel cup or pads in the shoe. • Calf muscles should be stretched after warm-up and cool-down.
Pain is at back of the heel Injury resembles Achilles tendonitis	Suspect **retrocalcaneal bursitis**: Treat the same as for Achilles tendonitis.
Pain, often disabling, is at bottom of the heel	Suspect **plantar fasciitis** ("heel spur"): • Apply ice for 20–30 minutes after activity and 3–4 times daily. • Use a heel cup in the shoe. • Reduce or stop activity. • Use an anti-inflammatory for 7 to 10 days.
Pain is in fifth metatarsal bone, possibly with swelling	Suspect **fracture** (Jones fracture): • Apply ice. • Stop activity. • Seek medical care.
Pain is on ball of foot between second and third toe	Suspect **Morton's neuroma:** • Wear wider, softer shoes. • If there is no improvement, surgery may be required.
Pain is on ball of foot at the big toe	Suspect **seasmoiditis or a stress fracture:** • Apply ice for 20–30 minutes, 3–4 times daily. • Rest. • Use an anti-inflammatory for 7 to 10 days. • If pain persists, seek medical care.
Area on skin has a "hot spot" (not very painful, red area) from rubbing	Suspect a **blister:** • Cool the hot spot with an ice pack. AND/OR • Tape several layers of moleskin, which are cut into a "doughnut-shape" to fit around the blister. OR • Apply duct-tape tightly over the painful area.
Blister is broken and fluid is seeping out	• Leave the "roof" on for protection. • Clean with soap and water. • Tape several layers of moleskin, cut into a "doughnut-shape" to fit around the blister. • Apply an antibiotic ointment in the hole over the blister. • Cover with an uncut gauze pad and tape in place.
Blister on foot is very painful, affects walking, and is not broken	• Drain the blister by puncturing the roof with several holes. • Leave the "roof" on for protection. • Clean with soap and water. • Tape several layers of moleskin, cut into a "doughnut-shape" to fit around the blister. • Apply an antibiotic ointment in the hole over the blister. • Place gauze pad over the moleskin and tape in place.

Table C.3	Determining and Treating Ankle Injuries (Ottawa Ankle Rules)
If...	**Then...**
Ankle is able to bear weight He/she is able to take four steps immediately after the injury and an hour later No tenderness or pain is felt when you push on the ankle knob bone	Suspect **ankle sprain:** • Use RICE procedures. • For the compression part of RICE, apply an elastic bandage over any soft pliable material (e.g., sock or t-shirt) placed in a "U" shape around the ankle knob with the curved part down. • Use an anti-inflammatory. • If pain and swelling do not decrease within 48 hours, seek medical care.
Ankle is unable to bear weight He/she is unable to take four steps immediately after the injury and an hour later Tenderness and pain is felt when you push on the ankle knob bone	Suspect **ankle fracture:** • Use RICE procedures. • For the compression part of RICE, apply an elastic bandage over any soft pliable material (e.g., sock or t-shirt) placed in a "U" shape around the ankle knob with the curved part down. • Use an anti-inflammatory. • Stabilize ankle against movement. • Seek medical care.

Table C.4	Determining and Treating Lower Leg Injuries
If...	**Then...**
Shin aches during activity, but: • Ache subsides significantly after activity stops • Ache is result of increase in workout routine (e.g., running longer, jogging on hills) • Shin is tender when pressed	Suspect **shin splints:** • Apply ice before activity and for 30 minutes after activity. • Stop activity until pain-free. • Use an anti-inflammatory.
Leg receives direct hit that produces: • Deformity, open wound, tenderness, and/or swelling	Suspect **fracture or bruise:** • Use RICE procedures. • Use an anti-inflammatory. • Control any bleeding. If fracture is suspected: • Stabilize leg against movement. • Seek medical care.
He/she feels a pop or sudden, sharp, burning pain in calf muscle while running or jumping	Suspect a **muscle strain** (tear, pull): • Use RICE procedures. • Use an anti-inflammatory.
He/she feels a pop while running or jumping causing pain just above the heel Leg is tender when pressed He/she is unable to bear weight on injured leg He/she has difficulty with controlling foot (flops around)	Suspect a **torn Achilles tendon:** • Use RICE procedures. • Use an anti-inflammatory. • Seek medical care.
A muscle (most often the calf muscle) goes into an uncontrolled spasm and contraction, resulting in severe pain and restriction or loss of movement	Suspect a **muscle cramp:** • Gently stretch the affected muscle, or • Relax the muscle by applying pressure to it. • Apply ice to the muscle. • Drink lightly salted cool water (dissolve ¼ teaspoon salt in a quart of water). Do not give salt tablets.

Knee

Knee injuries are among the most serious joint injuries **Table C.5**. Their severity is difficult to determine, thus you should seek medical care.

Thigh

The thigh consists of a single bone, the femur, which is surrounded and protected by heavy muscle. The muscle group on the front of the thigh is the "quadriceps." Most thigh injuries are from direct hits. Like with other leg muscles, a quadriceps strain can happen. See **Table C.6**.

Table C.5	Determining and Treating Knee Injuries
If...	**Then...**
Immediate swelling after injury Knee locks Knee gives way Pain occurs below kneecap Pain under the kneecap when climbing stairs	Suspect **knee injury** (acute and/or chronic): • Use RICE procedures. • Stabilize knee against movement. • Use an anti-inflammatory. • Seek medical care.
Examining for an acute injury (not overuse type of injury): **Pittsburgh Knee Rules:** Any blunt trauma or fall type injury and one of the following present: • Age younger than 12 years or over 50 years • Inability to walk four weight-bearing steps OR **Ottawa Knee Rules:** • Age over 55 years • Tenderness at the patella (kneecap) • Tenderness at head of fibula (bony knob on outside of knee) • Inability to flex knee to 90° • Inability to bear weight and take four steps immediately after injury and later	Suspect serious **knee injury**: • Use RICE procedures. • Stabilize knee against movement. • Use an anti-inflammatory. • Seek medical care.
Deformity obvious, with the kneecap (patella) on the outside (lateral side) of the knee. Compare it with the other kneecap.	Suspect a **dislocated kneecap**: • Apply ice. • Stabilize against movement. • Seek medical care.

Table C.6	Determining and Treating Thigh Injuries
If...	**Then...**
Pain at front of thigh	Suspect a **bruise:** • Use RICE procedures. • Use an anti-inflammatory.
Pain at back of thigh	Suspect a **muscle strain** (pulled hamstring): • Use RICE procedures. • Use an anti-inflammatory.

Hip

See ⬤ Table C.7 ⬤ to determine and treat hip injuries.

Finger

Most finger injures are not severe, but in rare cases a finger can dislocate—producing a grotesque deformity that requires immediate medical care. See ⬤ Table C.8 ⬤.

Elbow

More often than not, elbow injuries are nagging nuisances; occasionally an elbow will be more seriously injured. Rarely will an elbow dislocate. See ⬤ Table C.9 ⬤.

Shoulder

Shoulder injuries can range from mild to those that pose medical emergencies ⬤ Table C.10 ⬤. A dislocated shoulder usually occurs during contact sports and requires immediate medical care. A shoulder dislocation can be confused with a shoulder separation. The key difference is that in separation the shoulder joint and upper arm remain mobile. In dislocation, the mobility is lost.

Table C.7	Determining and Treating Hip Injuries
If...	**Then...**
Pain is in groin	Suspect **muscle strain:** • Use RICE procedures. • Use an anti-inflammatory.
Pain is on upper hip	Suspect **hip pointer:** • Use RICE procedures. • Use an anti-inflammatory.
Pain is on outer thigh to knee	Suspect **muscle strain or bursitis:** • Use RICE procedures. • Use an anti-inflammatory.

Table C.8	Determining and Treating Finger Injuries
If...	**Then...**

Deformed
Tender/painful
Swollen
	Suspect a possible **fracture and/or dislocation:**
	• Test for a finger fracture:
	  – If possible, straighten the fingers and place them flat on a hard surface.
	  – Tap the tip of the injured finger toward the hand. Pain lower down in the finger or into the hand can indicate a fracture.
	• Do **not** try to realign a dislocation.
	• Apply ice.
	• Stablize finger against movement by "buddy" taping for support.
	Or
	• Keeping hand and fingers in cupping shape as though holding a baseball with extra padding in the palm, secure the hand, fingers, and arm to a rigid board or folded newspapers.
	• Seek medical care.

C

Table C.9 — Determining and Treating Elbow Injuries

If...	Then...
Severe elbow pain after fall on arm	Suspect **dislocation or fracture:** • Apply ice. • Give an anti-inflammatory. • Stabilize against movement. • Seek medical care.
Elbow pain on inside (medial)	Suspect **"little league's, golfer's, or racquetball's" elbow:** • Use RICE procedures. • Give an anti-inflammatory. • Seek medical care if pain persists.
Elbow pain on outside (lateral)	Suspect **"tennis" elbow:** • Use RICE procedures. • Give an anti-inflammatory. • Seek medical care if pain persists.
Elbow with: • Tender/pain • Swelling	Suspect a **bruise:** • Use RICE procedures. • Seek medical care if tingling and/or weakness continue for 24 hours (can be serious because of possible nerve injury).

Table C.10 — Determining and Treating Shoulder Injuries

If...	Then...
Pain is on top of shoulder after a fall or being hit	Suspect a **separation:** • Apply ice. • Use an anti-inflammatory. • Seek medical care.
Extreme pain is at front of shoulder after a fall Victim holds upper arm away from the body, supported by the uninjured arm Arm cannot be brought across the chest to touch the opposite shoulder Victim describes a history of previous dislocations	Suspect a **dislocation:** • Apply ice. • Stabilize shoulder against movement and immediately seek medical care.
Burning pain is felt down arm after twisting neck	Suspect a **"stinger":** • Apply ice. • Use an anti-inflammatory. • Seek medical care.
Arm goes limp	Suspect a **subluxation:** • Apply ice. • Use an anti-inflammatory. • Seek medical care.
Pain is felt when raising arm	Suspect a **rotor cuff:** • Apply ice. • Use an anti-inflammatory. • Seek medical care.

Muscle

See [Table C.11] to determine and treat muscle injuries.

Chest

See [Table C.12] for symptoms and treatment of chest injuries.

Breathing Difficulty

See [Table C.13] to determine and treat breathing difficulty.

Table C.11 — Determining and Treating Muscle Injuries

If...	Then...
Muscle pain occurs 12 to 72+ hours after physical activity	Suspect **delayed-onset muscle soreness:** • Apply ice (some experts suggest heat). • Warm up. • Stretch the muscle. • Do not use nonsteriodial medications (e.g., ibuprofen, aspirin).

Table C.12 — Determining and Treating Chest Injuries

If...	Then...
Sudden, severe central chest pain: • Can occur at rest • Worse when exerting • Pain is crushing, vice-like • May radiate up to the jaws or down the left arm Nausea Breathlessness Sweating Blueness of lips	Suspect a **heart attack:** 1. Give one aspirin to chew (not any other analgesic, only aspirin). 2. Seek medical care immediately—usually by calling 9-1-1. 3. Monitor for possible cardiac arrest requiring CPR. 4. Help victim into least painful position—usually sitting with legs bent at the knees. 5. Ask if he or she is taking a medication known as nitroglycerin; if so, help person take it.
No chest pain, but: Sudden general tiredness Breathlessness as a new symptom Sudden worsening of existing breathlessness	Suspect a **silent heart attack:** • Treat as you would a heart attack.

Table C.13 — Determining and Treating Breathing Difficulty

If...	Then...
Coughing Wheezing, especially when breathing out Chest feels "tight" Sweating, breathless, rapid pulse Neck muscles strain in an attempt to increase breathing As attack worsens, blue lips, tiredness, drowsiness Confusion, coma Poor response to usual medication	Suspect **asthma** (asthma can be induced during exercise): 1. Place victim in a comfortable, upright position to help breathing. 2. Help victim use medicines (inhaler and/or pills). 3. Give plenty of fluids. 4. Seek medical care if: • No improvement within 2 hours after using medications. • There are repeated attacks. • Attack is severe and prolonged.

C

How Heat Affects the Body

Human bodies dissipate heat by varying the rate and depth of blood circulation, by losing water through the skin and sweat glands, and—when blood is heated above 98.6°F —by panting. The heart begins to pump more blood, blood vessels dilate to accommodate the increased flow, and the bundles of tiny capillaries threading through the upper layers of skin are put into operation. The body's blood is circulated closer to the skin's surface, and excess heat drains off into the cooler atmosphere. At the same time, water diffuses through the skin as perspiration. The skin handles about 90% of the body's heat dissipating function.

Sweating, on its own, does nothing to cool the body, unless the water is removed by evaporation—and high relative humidity retards evaporation. The evaporation process works this way: the heat energy required to evaporate sweat is extracted from the body, thereby cooling it. Under conditions of high temperature (above 90°F) and high relative humidity, the body is doing everything it can to maintain an internal temperature of 98.6°F. The heart is pumping a torrent of blood through dilated circulatory vessels; the sweat glands are pouring liquid—including essential dissolved chemicals, like sodium and chloride—onto the surface of the skin.

Too Much Heat

Heat disorders generally occur from a reduction or collapse of the body's ability to shed heat by circulatory changes and sweating, or a chemical (salt) imbalance caused by too much sweating. When heat gain exceeds the level the body can remove, or when the body cannot compensate for fluids and salt lost through perspiration, the temperature of the body's inner core begins to rise and heat-related illness may develop.

Heat illnesses include a range of disorders **Table C.14**. Some of them are common, but only heatstroke is life threatening. Untreated heatstroke victims always die.

Ranging in severity, heat disorders share one common feature: the individual has been overexposed or has overexercised for his or her age and physical condition in the existing thermal environment.

Studies indicate that, other factors being equal, the severity of heat disorders tend to increase with age—heat cramps in a 17-year-old may be heat exhaustion in someone 40, and heat stroke in a person over 60.

Acclimatization concerns adjusting sweat–salt concentration, among other things. The idea is to lose enough water to regulate body temperature, with the least possible chemical disturbance.

Heat index (or apparent temperature) is how the heat and humidity in the air combine to make us feel **Figure C.1**. Higher humidity plus higher temperatures often combine to make us feel a perceived temperature that is higher than the actual air temperature. The old saying, "it's not the heat, it's the humidity," holds true.

The National Weather Service is using a new "mean heat index" to alert people to the dangers of heat waves. The index, which went into use in May 2002, measures how hot a person will feel over a full day.

The idea is the same as the traditional heat index, which shows how hot a particular combination of heat and humidity feels. This index has usually been used to show the danger during the hottest part of the day.

The mean heat index averages the heat index from the hottest and coolest parts of a day.

Table C.14 — Determining and Treating Heat-Related Illnesses

If...	Then...

Skin is extremely hot when touched—usually dry, but may be moist
Altered mental status, ranging from slight confusion, agitation, and disorientation to unresponsiveness
	Suspect **heatstroke:**
	Heatstoke is life-threatening and must be treated immediately.
	1. Move victim to a cool place. Monitor ABCs.
	2. Remove clothing down to victim's underwear.
	3. Keep victim's head and shoulders slightly raised.
	4. Quickly cool the victim:
	  • Spray the victim with water and vigorously fan. This method does not work well in high humidity.
	  • If ice is available, place ice packs into the armpits, sides of the neck, and groin.
	5. Stop cooling when mental status improves or if shivering occurs.
	6. Evacuate to medical care ASAP. Continue cooling during evacuation.

Sweating Thirsty Fatigued Flu-like symptoms—headache, nausea Shortness of breath Rapid pulse Differences from heatstroke: • No altered mental status • Skin is not hot, but clammy	Suspect **heat exhaustion:** Uncontrolled heat exhaustion can evolve into heatstroke. 1. Move victim to a cool place. 2. Have the victim remove excess clothing. 3. Have the victim drink cool fluids. 4. For more severe cases, give lightly salted cool water (dissolve $\frac{1}{4}$ teaspoon salt in a quart of water). Do not give salt tablets. 5. Raise victim's legs 8" to 12" (keep legs straight). 4. Cool the victim, but not as aggressively as for heatstroke. 5. If no improvement is seen within 30 minutes, seek medical care.
Painful muscle spasms that happen suddenly Affects muscle in the back of the leg or abdominal muscles Occurs during or after physical exertion	Suspect **heat cramp:** Relief may take several hours. 1. Rest in a cool area. 2. Drink lightly salted cool water (dissolve $\frac{1}{4}$ teaspoon salt in 1 quart of water) or a commercial sports drink. Do not give salt tablets. 3. Stretch the cramped calf muscle or try acupressure method of pinching the upper lip just below the nose.
Victim is dizzy or faints	Suspect **heat syncope:** 1. If unresponsive, check ABCs. Person usually recovers quickly. 2. If victim fell, check for injuries. 2. Have victim rest and lie down with legs raised in cool area. 4. Wet skin by splashing water on face. 3. If not nauseated, drink lightly salted cool water (dissolve $\frac{1}{4}$ teaspoon salt in 1 quart of water) or a commercial sports drink. Do not give salt tablets.
Ankles and feet swell Occurs during first few days in a hot environment	Suspect **heat edema:** 1. Wear support stockings. 2. Elevate legs.
Itchy rash on skin wet from sweating	Suspect **prickly heat:** 1. Dry and cool skin. 2. Limit heat exposure.

C

Relative Humidity (%)

°F	40	45	50	55	60	65	70	75	80	85	90	95	100
110	136												
108	130	137											
106	124	130	137										
104	119	124	131	137									
102	114	119	124	130	137								
100	109	114	118	124	139	136							
98	106	109	113	117	123	128	134						
96	101	104	108	112	116	121	126	132					
94	97	100	101	106	110	114	118	124	129	135			
92	94	96	99	101	105	108	112	116	121	125	131		
90	91	93	95	97	100	103	106	109	113	117	122	127	132
88	88	89	91	93	95	98	100	100	106	110	113	114	121
86	85	87	88	89	91	93	95	97	100	102	105	108	112
84	83	84	85	86	88	89	90	92	94	96	98	100	103
82	81	82	83	84	84	85	86	88	89	90	91	93	95
80	80	80	81	81	82	82	83	84	84	85	86	86	87

Air Temperature

Heat Index
(Apparent
Temperature)

With Prolonged Exposure
and/or Physical Activity

Extreme Danger

Heat stroke or sunstroke
highly likely

Danger

Sunstroke, muscle cramps,
and/or heat exhaustion likely

Extreme Caution

Sunstroke, muscle cramps,
and/or heat exhaustion possible

Caution

Fatigue possible

Figure C.1

The heat index (or apparent temperature) shows how heat and humidity affect the human body.
(*Source:* National Weather Service. http//www.crh.noaa.gov/ict/heat.htm.)

Sunburn

Sunburn, with its ultraviolet radiation burns, can significantly retard the skin's ability to
shed excess heat.

See **Table C.15** to determine and treat sunburns.

Table C.15	Determining and Treating Sunburns
If...	**Then...**
Skin that has been exposed to the sun later becomes: • red • mildly swollen • tender and painful	Suspect **first-degree (superficial) sunburn:** 1. Immerse burned area in cold water or by applying a wet, cold cloth until pain-free, both in and out of the water (usually 10–45 min.). If cold water is unavailable, use any cold liquid available. 2. Give ibuprofen (for children, give acetaminophen). 3. Have victim drink as much water as possible without becoming nauseous. 4. Keep burned arm or leg raised. 5. After burn has been cooled, apply aloe vera gel or inexpensive moisturizer. First-degree burns do **not** have to covered.

Skin that has been exposed to the sun later becomes:
• blistered
• swollen
• weeping of fluids
• severely painful
	Suspect **second-degree (partial thickness) sunburn:**
	• If skin affected is less than 20% body surface (victim's palm, not including fingers and thumb, equals 1% of body surface area):
	  1. Follow same procedures (steps 1–4) as for a first-degree burn, with these additions:
	  2. After burn has been cooled, apply thin layer of antibacterial ointment (eg., bacitracin, Neosporin®)
	  3. Cover burn with a dry, nonsticking, sterile dressing or clean cloth.
	• If skin has a large second-degree burn over more than 20% of the body surface area:
	  1. Follow steps 2–4 of first-degree burn care.
	  2. Seek medical care.
	    Do **not** apply cold because it may cause hypothermia.

Cold-related Injuries

Hypothermia

Hypothermia happens when the body's temperature (98.6°F, 37°C) drops more than 2° **Table C.16**. Hypothermia does not require subfreezing temperatures. Severe hypothermia is life-threatening. Check also for possible frostbite.

Table C.16	Determining and Treating Hypothermia
If...	**Then...**

Shivering uncontrollably
Has the "umbles"—grumbles, mumbles, fumbles, and stumbles
Has cool abdomen when felt with a warm hand
	Suspect **mild hypothermia:**
	1. Stop heat loss:
	  • Get victim out of the cold.
	  • Handle victim gently.
	  • Replace wet clothing with dry clothing.
	  • Add insulation (e.g., blankets, towels, pillows, sleeping bags) beneath and around victim. Cover victim's head (50–80% of body's heat loss is through the head).
	2. Keep in flat (horizontal) position.
	3. Allow the victim to shiver—do not stop the shivering by adding heat. Shivering, which generates heat, will rewarm mildly hypothermic victims. DO NOT use the following procedures because they stop shivering:
	  • Warm water immersion.
	  • Body-to-body contact.
	  • Chemical heat pads.
	Warm drinks are unable to rewarm sufficiently. However, warm sugary liquids can provide calories for shivering to continue and may provide a psychological boost.
	DO NOT give alcohol to drink.

Muscles are rigid and stiff No shivering Skin feels ice cold and appears blue Altered mental status Slow pulse Slow breathing Victim appears to be dead	Suspect **severe hypothermia:** 1. Follow steps 1 and 2 from mild hypothermia for all hypothermic victims. 2. Check ABCs and give CPR as necessary. Check the pulse for 30 to 45 seconds before starting CPR. 3. Gently evacuate victim to medical help for rewarming. Rewarming in a remote location is difficult and rarely effective. However, when the victim is far from medical care, the victim must be warmed by any available external heat source (e.g., body-to body contact, warm water immersion).

C

Frostbite and Frostnip

Frostbite happens only in below freezing temperatures (<32°F) (Figure C.2). Mainly the feet, hands, ears, and nose are affected. The most severe results are gangrene requiring surgical amputation. See (Table C.17) for symptoms and treatment. Check for hypothermia, since it may also be present.

Frostnip is caused when water on the skin's surface freezes (Table C.18).

Wind Chill Chart

Wind (mph)

Calm	5	10	15	20	25	30	35	40	45	50	55	60
40	36	34	32	30	29	28	28	27	26	26	25	25
35	31	27	25	24	23	22	21	20	19	19	18	17
30	25	21	19	17	16	15	14	13	12	12	11	10
25	19	15	13	11	9	8	7	6	5	4	4	3
20	13	9	6	4	3	1	0	−1	−2	−3	−3	−4
15	7	3	0	−2	−4	−5	−7	−8	−9	−10	−11	−11
10	1	−4	−7	−9	−11	−12	−14	−15	−16	−17	−18	−19
5	−5	−10	−13	−15	−17	−19	−21	−22	−23	−24	−25	−26
0	−11	−16	−19	−22	−24	−26	−27	−29	−30	−31	−32	−33
−5	−16	−22	−26	−29	−31	−33	−34	−36	−37	−38	−39	−40
−10	−22	−28	−32	−35	−37	−39	−41	−43	−44	−45	−46	−48
−15	−28	−35	−39	−42	−44	−46	−48	−50	−51	−52	−54	−55
−20	−34	−41	−45	−48	−51	−53	−55	−57	−58	−60	−61	−62
−25	−40	−47	−51	−55	−58	−60	−62	−64	−65	−67	−68	−69
−30	−46	−53	−58	−61	−64	−67	−69	−71	−72	−74	−75	−76
−35	−52	−59	−64	−68	−71	−73	−76	−78	−79	−81	−82	−84
−40	−57	−66	−71	−74	−78	−80	−82	−84	−86	−88	−89	−91
−45	−63	−72	−77	−81	−84	−87	−89	−91	−93	−95	−97	−98

Temperature (°F)

Note: Frostbite occurs in 15 minutes or less.

$$\text{Wind Chill (°F)} = 35.74 + 0.6215T - 35.75(V^{0.16}) + 0.4275T(V^{0.16})$$

Where, T = Air Temperature (°F)
V = Wind Speed (mph)

Figure C.2

Wind chill chart. (*Source:* National Weather Service. http://www.erh.noaa.gov/er/iln/tables.htm.)

Table C.17 — Determining and Treating Frostbite

If...	Then...	
Skin color is white, waxy, or grayish-yellow Affected part is cold and numb Tingling, stinging, or aching sensation is felt Skin surface feels stiff or crusty, and underlying tissue feels soft when depressed gently	Suspect **superficial frostbite:**	All frostbite injuries require the same first aid treatment: 1. Get victim to a warm area. 2. Replace wet clothing or constricting items that could impair blood circulation (e.g., rings). 3. Do not rub or massage the area. 4. For deep frostbite, seek medical care. 5. When more than 1 hour from medical facility, place part in warm water (test by pouring some over the inside of your arm to test that it is warm, not hot). For ear or face, it is best but may be difficult to apply warm moist cloths, changing them frequently. May have to cover with warm hands. Give pain medication (preferable aspirin or ibuprofen). Rewarming may take 20 to 40 minutes or when parts become soft. **DO NOT:** • Rub or massage part. • Rewarm w/ stove, vehicle's tailpipe exhaust, or over a fire. • Break blisters.
Affected part feels cold, hard, and solid, and cannot be depressed—feels like a piece of wood or frozen meat Affected part is pale, and skin may appear waxy A painfully cold part suddenly stops hurting Blisters appear after rewarming	Suspect **deep frostbite:**	• Allow victim to smoke or drink alcohol. • Rewarm if there is any possibility of refreezing. • Allow thawed part to refreeze. After thawing: • Place dry, sterile gauze between toes and fingers to prevent sticking. • Elevate part to reduce pain and swelling. • Give aspirin or ibuprofen for pain and inflammation. Do not give to children. • Apply thin layer of aloe vera on area. • Seek medical care.

Table C.18 — Determining and Treating Frostnip

If...	Then...
Skin appears red and sometimes swollen Painful	Suspect **frostnip:** (It is difficult to tell the difference between frostnip and frostbite.): 1. Gently warm area against a warm body part (e.g., armpit, stomach, bare hands) or by blowing warm air on the area. 2. Do not rub area.

Knowledge Check and Critical Thinking Answer Key

Chapter 1 Changing to a Healthy Lifestyle

Knowledge Check
1. B
2. D
3. D

Critical Thinking
1. C
2. C
3. B

Chapter 2 Preparing for Physical Activity and Exercise

Knowledge Check
1. D
2. B
3. C

Critical Thinking
1. A
2. B
3. C

Chapter 3 Improving Cardiorespiratory Endurance

Knowledge Check
1. A
2. B
3. B

Critical Thinking
1. A
2. C
3. B

Chapter 4 Increasing Flexibility

Knowledge Check
1. A
2. B
3. C

Critical Thinking
1. A
2. B
3. A
4. A

Chapter 5 Increasing Muscular Strength and Endurance

Knowledge Check
1. C
2. B
3. D

Critical Thinking
1. B
2. B
3. B
4. B
5. C

Chapter 6 Choosing a Nutritious Diet

Knowledge Check
1. B
2. C
3. C

Critical Thinking
1. A
2. A
3. A
4. A
5. C
6. D

D

Chapter 7   Assessing Body Composition

Knowledge Check

1. A
2. C
3. C

Critical Thinking

1. A
2. B
3. C
4. C

Chapter 8   Maintaining a Healthy Body Composition and Body Weight

Knowledge Check

1. A
2. C
3. B

Critical Thinking

1. B
2. C
3. C
4. C
5. A

Chapter 9   Managing Stress

Knowledge Check

1. A
2. E
3. C

Critical Thinking

1. A
2. C
3. D
4. A

Chapter 10   Making Informed Choices

Knowledge Check

1. B
2. C
3. A

Critical Thinking

1. B
2. A
3. B

Glossary

A

adenosine triphosphate (ATP) The only useable form of energy used in the human body.

adrenaline A hormone that prepares the body to react during times of stress or in an emergency.

aerobic exercise Exercise that depends on oxygen for energy production.

aerobic energy system System that needs oxygen to produce energy.

allostatic load The ongoing demand on the body from long-term exposure to stress hormones.

amenorrhea Absence of normal menstruation.

anabolic steroids Synthetic male hormones that increase muscle size and strength.

anaerobic Without using oxygen.

anaerobic energy system System that creates energy for activities that last less than five minutes or have frequent rest periods.

anemia A reduction in the number of red blood cells in the blood. Anemia is not a disease but a symptom of various diseases, including iron deficiency.

anorexia nervosa Extreme restriction of food intake.

antioxidants A substance that can combine with or neutralize free radicals, and thus prevent oxidative damage to cells and tissues.

asanas Various postures used in doing yoga exercises.

atrophy Shrinkage of fat or muscle.

autonomic nervous system Part of the nervous system that controls automatic body functions, such as blood pressure, heart rate, and breathing. Subdivided into sympathetic and parasympathetic.

B

ballistic stretching Bouncing, repetitive movement during stretching.

basal metabolic rate (BMR) Energy consumed (measured in calories) by the body at rest to keep vital functions going.

binge eating Uncontrolled eating during a short time period.

bioelectrical impedance Measurement of the strength and speed of an electrical signal sent through the body.

blaming Placing the responsibility of an unmet goal on someone else.

body composition Proportion of fat, muscle, bone, and other tissues in the body.

body mass index (BMI) A measure of body fatness, calculated by dividing your weight in pounds by your height in inches. Then divide that answer by your height in inches. Multiply by 703.

botulism Poisoning by the toxin of the microorganism *Clostridium botulinum*.

bulimia Periodic bingeing followed by purging, or alternate days of bingeing and fasting.

C

calorie Unit of energy supplied by food; equals 1 kilocalorie (1 kcal), the amount if heated required to raise the temperature of 1 kilo of water 1°C.

carbo loading Stuffing yourself with complex carbohydrates during the days before an endurance event.

carbohydrates Nutrient that is the body's main source of energy; consists of sugars and starches found in grains, vegetables, and fruits; two types are simple and complex.

cardiorespiratory endurance activity Exercise that contracts large muscle groups and increases breathing and heart rate.

cellulite Adipose tissue surrounded by stretched connective tissue.

cholesterol Wax-like substance made by the body's liver and found in animal and plant foods.

collars Devices used to secure weights to a barbell or dumbbell. Without collars the weights on one side of the bar will slip off.

complete protein Contains all the essential amino acids.

consistency The constant activity level needed to maintain fitness.

contusions Bruising of tissue.

cool-down The 5–10 minutes at the end of a workout involving light movement and stretching.

CPR (cardiopulmonary resuscitation) Clearing air passages to the lungs, giving mouth-to-mouth respiration, and massaging the heart to restore normal breathing after cardiac arrest.

cramping Muscular tightness and abdominal or limb pain from dehydration and high body temperature.

creatine phosphate (CP) Chemical present in muscles that makes ATP rapidly for thirty seconds' worth of exercise. Creatine phosphate is produced in the body from the digestion of meat. It can also be found as a supplement. Research is inconclusive as to its benefits or long-term risks.

cross-training Combining the components of fitness in a workout program, instead of focusing on only one area.

D

dietary fiber Nondigestible carbohydrates found in plants; two types are soluble and insoluble.

dislocations Bones are displaced from their normal joint alignment, out of their sockets, or out of their normal positions.

distress Harmful or bad response to a stressor.

dynamic or active stretching Muscle is taken beyond its normal range of motion with help from a partner.

E

eating disorder A spectrum of abnormal eating patterns that eventually may endanger a person's health or increase the risk for other diseases. Generally, psychological factors play a key role.

endocrine system Consists of glands that produce hormones that control body functions.

endorphins Protein produced in your brain that serves as your body's natural painkiller. Endorphins also reduce stress, depression, and anxiety.

endurance Ability to work out for a period of time without fatigue.

essential amino acids The nine protein amino acids that the body cannot make, and therefore, must come from foods you eat.

essential body fat Minimum amount of body fat needed for good health.

eustress Helpful or good response to a stressor.

exercise Planned, structured, and repetitive physical activity done to improve or maintain one or more components of physical fitness.

exercise log A record of your activity that includes the type, duration, and intensity of each exercise each day.

F

female athlete triad Combination of eating disorders, amenorrhea, and osteoporosis.

fitness The body's response to physical effort.

flexibility Ability to move a joint smoothly through a full range of motion.

free radicals A short-lived chemical that can have detrimental effects on cells.

frequency How often; the number of times an exercise or group of exercises is performed within a certain time frame.

G

general adaptation syndrome A series of body changes that result from stress. The syndrome occurs in three stages: alarm, resistance, and exhaustion.

genetic modification Manipulating the DNA of an organism to change some of its characteristics.

gland A group of cells that secretes hormones.

glucose Simple sugar circulating in the blood.

glycogen Complex carbohydrates stored primarily in the skeletal muscles and liver. When energy is needed, glycogen is converted to glucose.

H

health The 1946 World Health Organization's definition of health has been used as a foundation for the contemporary term of wellness. "Health is a state of complete physical, mental, and social well-being and not merely the absence of disease or infirmity."

high-density lipoprotein (HDL) Carries cholesterol from the blood back to the liver which processes the cholesterol for elimination from the body. It is often referred to as the *good* cholesterol.

homeostasis Stability and consistency of a person's physiology.

hormone Chemical messenger released into the bloodstream that controls many body activities.

hydrostatic weighing Measuring a person's weight while he or she is suspended in water.

hypertrophy Enlargement of fat or muscle.

I

immediate energy system System using existing cellular ATP during first 10 seconds of activity.

incomplete protein A protein lacking one or more of the essential amino acids.

individual differences The variables in our physical ability.

insoluble fiber Does not dissolve in water.

intensity The amount of energy exerted while performing an exercise.

irradiation Treatment with gamma rays, X rays, or high-voltage electrons to kill pathogens and, in the case of food, to increase shelf life.

L

lactic acid Chemical formed when muscles must use stored glucose or blood sugar to produce ATP.

lacto-ovo-vegetarian Person who includes milk, dairy products, and eggs in his or her diet.

lacto-vegetarian Person who includes some or all dairy products in his or her diet.

lipids Fats or fatlike substances characterized by their insolubility in water or solubility in fat.

lipoprotein Allows cholesterol to dissolve in the blood and carries it through the bloodstream to all parts of the body; two main types are high-density lipoprotein (HDL) and low-density lipoprotein (LDL).

locus of control The figurative place where a person locates the source of responsibility for the events in his or her life.

lordosis Excessive pelvic tilt.

low-density lipoprotein (LDL) Carries cholesterol from the liver to the rest of the body. When there is too much LDL cholesterol in the blood, it can be deposited on the walls of the coronary arteries. It is often referred to as the *bad* cholesterol.

M

macrominerals Minerals needed by the body in amounts greater than 100 mg.

macronutrients Nutrients needed by your body in relatively large amounts.

mall-walking Walking a circuit around the lobby floors of an enclosed shopping mall in the morning before the stores open.

maximal oxygen uptake ($VO_{2\,max}$) How efficiently the cardiorespiratory system uses oxygen.

metabolism The rate at which your body uses energy.

microminerals or trace minerals Minerals needed by the body in amounts less than 100 mg.

micronutrients Nutrients needed by your body in relatively small amounts.

minerals Inorganic nutrients that regulate many chemical reactions in the body.

monounsaturated High concentrations of unsaturated fat in canola, peanut, and olive oils.

motivation The underlying drive behind making changes.

multiple-joint exercise An exercise in which two or more joints move together.

muscular endurance The ability of muscles to apply force repeatedly.

muscular strength The force muscles can exert against resistance.

N

nutrients Substances in food the body needs for normal function and good health.

O

obesity Excessive amounts of body fat.

osteoporosis Disease related to calcium deficiency in which bones become thin and brittle and fracture easily.

overload Placing a greater-than-normal amount of stress (within reason) on the body in order to make it function at a higher capacity.

P

pathogens Microorganisms causing disease.

pH (powerHydrogen) Condition of a solution represented by a number on a scale of acidity to alkalinity.

physical activity Bodily movement produced by skeletal muscles that increases energy expenditure.

physical fitness Set of attributes that people have or achieve that relates to the ability to perform physical activity.

phytochemical Substance in plants (*phyto* = plant) that may have beneficial effects on the body.

polyunsaturated High concentrations of unsaturated fat in sunflower, corn, soybean oils, and fish.

procrastination Pushing a task to a later point in time.

progression The gradual increase of the level and intensity of exercise.

progressive muscular relaxation Systematically tensing and relaxing the body's muscles from the feet to the head.

progressive overloading Increasing, from one session to another, the amount of weight you lift during a set.

protein Nutrient made up of amino acids that is needed for growth to build, repair, and maintain body tissues.

psychoneuroimmunology Study of nervous, endocrine, and immune system interaction.

pulmonary circulation Circulation between the heart and the lungs.

pulse The surge of blood that can be felt on certain points on the body each time the heart pumps blood into the arteries.

R

rate of perceived exertion A person's own perception of the intensity of his or her exercise.

rationalization Making excuses for not carrying out a task.

relaxation response Reversal of stress symptoms.

repetition (rep) A single lifting and lowering of the weight.

repetition maximums The maximum weight you can lift successfully once while using proper form.

resistance training Building muscle by working against the resistance of weights.

rest A period of inactivity to allow your body to recover from strenuous exercise.

reversibility The principle that states that the results of physical fitness are not permanent.

S

safety Awareness of all aspects of your exercise routine to protect yourself from injury.

saturated fat Fat from meat, poultry, dairy products, and hardened vegetable fat.

semi or partial vegetarian Person who eats no red meat, but may include chicken or fish, dairy products, and eggs in his or her diet.

set Number of reps performed without stopping to rest.

soluble fiber Partially dissolves in water.

specificity The type of physical changes you desire in your body relates directly to the type of exercise you choose.

spotter Another person who can help if the weight tilts or can help move a weight into position before or after a lift.

sprains Tearing or stretching of the joints that causes mild to severe damage to the ligaments and joint capsules.

static or passive stretching Muscle is stretched naturally without force being applied.

storage fat Fat deposited in adipose tissue (fat cells) that protects organs and insulates the body.

strains Muscles are stretched or torn.

stress The physical and emotional tension that comes from situations the body perceives as threatening.

stressor A source or cause of stress, may be physical, mental, social, or environmental.

stretch reflex An involuntary muscle contraction against a quick stretch.

stretching Primary method of improving flexibility.

sympathetic nervous system Subsystem of the autonomic system that triggers your body's response to stress—known as the fight-or-flight response.

systemic circulation Circulation between the heart and the rest of the body.

T

t'ai chi Thirteenth-century Chinese exercise routine involving graceful dancelike movements.

target heart rate zone A range of heart rates used to maintain optimal effects during aerobic exercise.

tendinitis Inflammation of a tendon from overuse.

time How long; the duration an exercise or group of exercises takes to complete.

trans fatty acids Fats produced by heating liquid vegetable oils in the presence of hydrogen. This process is called hydrogenation.

type The classification of exercise.

Type 2 Diabetes A disease that involves the inability to produce an adequate amount of insulin.

type A An individual exhibiting a sense of time urgency ("hurry sickness"), aggressiveness, and competitiveness, usually combined with hostility. Describes a great majority of Americans.

type B An individual displaying no sense of time urgency, no hostility, noncompetitiveness, patience, and a secure sense of self-esteem.

U

underweight A BMI under 19.

unsaturated fat Type of fat obtained from plant sources and fish; two types are monounsaturated and polyunsaturated.

V

vegan Person who eats only foods of plant origin.

vegetarian diet Diet in which vegetables are the foundation and meat products are restricted or eliminated.

vitamin Nutrient necessary for normal functioning of the body; two types are water-soluble and fat-soluble.

VO_{2max} Amount of oxygen the body uses when it reaches its maximum ability to supply oxygen during exercise.

W

warm-up The 5–10 minutes of low-intensity movement at the beginning of a workout that prepares the body for activity by increasing muscle temperature and metabolism.

wasting Occurs when the diet lacks protein; the body breaks down body tissue (e.g., muscle) and uses it as a protein source.

weight management The adoption of healthful and sustainable eating and exercise behaviors indicated for reduced disease risk and improved feelings of energy and well-being.

wellness The National Wellness Institute offers that wellness is an active process of becoming aware of and making choices toward a more successful existence.

Index

Photo Credits

Unless otherwise acknowledged, all photos are the property of Jones and Bartlett Publishers.

p. ii, © image100/Alamy Images; p. v, © AbleStock; p. vi, © LiquidLibrary; p. vii, © (top) LiquidLibrary; p. viii, (top) PhotoDisc; p. ix, © PhotoDisc; p. x, Courtesy of Bill Branson/National Cancer Institute; p. xi, © LiquidLibrary; p. xii, © Thinkstock/Index Stock Imagery; p. xiii, © Photos.com; p. xiv, © Photos.com; p. xvii, © Ryan McVay/PhotoDisc/ Getty Images; p. xviii, © Photos.com; p. xix, © PhotoDisc; p. xx, © Keith Brofsky/PhotoDisc/ Getty Images; p. xxii, © PhotoDisc; p. 1, © AbleStock; p. 3, © PhotoDisc; p. 5, © Photos.com; p. 6, © Ryan McVay/PhotoDisc; p. 8, © Ryan McVay/PhotoDisc; p. 11, © LiquidLibrary; p. 12, © Photos.com; p. 16, © Ron Chapple/Thinkstock/ Alamy Images; p. 17, © LiquidLibrary; p. 18, (top) © Donna Day/Stone/Getty Images, (bottom) © LiquidLibrary; p. 19, (top) © AbleStock, (bottom) © LiquidLibrary; p. 20, © LiquidLibrary; p. 21, © Ryan McVay/PhotoDisc; p. 23, (top) © Karl Weatherly/PhotoDisc/Getty Images, (middle) © AbleStock, (bottom) © LiquidLibrary; p. 24, © Polo Productions/BrandX Pictures/Alamy Images; p. 25, © AbleStock; p. 26, © AbleStock; p. 30, © LiquidLibrary; p. 32, © Robert Brenner/ PhotoEdit; p. 35, (top) © PhotoDisc, (bottom) © Frank Siteman/PhotoEdit; p. 37, © PhotoDisc; p. 39, © PhotoDisc/Getty Images; p. 41, (top) © Photos.com, (middle), © LiquidLibrary, (bottom) © LiquidLibrary; p. 42, (top) © E. Dygas/PhotoDisc, (middle) © LiquidLibrary, (bottom) © AbleStock; p. 43, (top) © LiquidLibrary, (bottom) © Keith Brofsky/PhotoDisc/Getty Images; p. 44, (top) © Luca DiCecco/Alamy Images, (bottom) © PhotoDisc; p. 50, © PhotoDisc; p. 52, © Photos.com; p. 55, Courtesy Danny Meyer/U.S. Air Force; p. 80, © SW Productions/PhotoDisc/Getty Images; p. 81, © LiquidLibrary; p. 84, © PhotoDisc; p. 85, © PhotoDisc; p. 86, (top) © Ryan McVay/PhotoDisc/ Getty Images, (bottom left) © Jess Alford/ PhotoDisc, (bottom middle) © Jules Frazier/ PhotoDisc, (bottom right) © Photolink/PhotoDisc;

p. 87, © PhotoDisc; p. 88, © PhotoDisc; p. 90, © AbleStock; p. 94, © LiquidLibrary; p. 95, © Ron Chapple/Thinkstock/Alamy Images; p. 96, (top) © AbleStock, (bottom) © AbleStock; p. 97, © LiquidLibrary; p. 105, © PhotoDisc; p. 107, (top) © Bill Aron/PhotoEdit, (bottom) © PhotoDisc; p. 110, © AbleStock; p. 113, © LiquidLibrary; p. 118, © Oscar Knott/FogStock/Alamy Images; p. 119, Courtesy of Bill Branson/National Cancer Institute; p. 121, (left) © Prado, Madrid, Spain/ The Bridgeman Art Library, (right) © Max Nash/ AP Photo; p. 123, (top) © David Young-Wolff/ PhotoEdit; p. 124, (top) © Life Measurement Instruments, (middle) © SPL/Custom Medical Stock Photo, (bottom) © SPL/Custom Medical Stock Photo; p. 130, © Rubberball Productions; p. 131, © LiquidLibrary; p. 134, © Robert W. Ginn/ PhotoEdit; p. 135, (top) © Ed Reschke, (bottom) © David Young-Wolff/PhotoEdit; p. 137, © Stock Connection Distribution/Alamy Images; p. 138, (top) David Young-Wolff/PhotoEdit, (bottom) © PhotoDisc; p. 139, (left) © PhotoDisc, (right) © AbleStock; p. 140, © AbleStock; p. 142, © John Bolivar/Custom Medical Stock Photo; p. 145, © PhotoDisc; p. 150, © John Foxx/Alamy Images; p. 151, © Thinkstock/Index Stock Imagery; p. 152, © AbleStock; p. 153, © LiquidLibrary; p. 154, (top) © Thinkstock/Getty Images, (bottom) © Sheila Terry/Science Source/Photo Researchers; p. 158, © Owen Frank/Stock Boston/PNI; p. 159, © Photos.com; p. 160, (top) © AbleStock, (middle) © Creatas, (bottom) © AbleStock; p. 161, © AbleStock; p. 162, © Photos.com; p. 163, © AbleStock; p. 164, Courtesy of Jacqueline Mark; p. 165, (top) © LiquidLibrary, (bottom) © Photos.com; p. 168, © PhotoDisc; p. 170 (top left) © LiquidLibrary, (top right) © Myrleen Ferguson Cate/PhotoEdit, (bottom) © LiquidLibrary; p. 171, (top) © Robert Brenner/PhotoEdit, (middle) © David Young-Wolff/PhotoEdit, (bottom) © AbleStock; p. 172, © Photos.com; p. 173, (top) © AbleStock, (bottom) © Photos.com; p. 174, © LiquidLibrary; p. 175, (top) © LiquidLibrary, (bottom) © Michael Newman/PhotoEdit.